The Physician's Essential MBA

What Every Physician Leader Needs to Know

Michael J. Stahl, PhD
Director, Physician Executive MBA
Distinguished Professor of Management
College of Business Administration
The University of Tennessee
Knoxville, Tennessee

Peter J. Dean, PhD
Associate Professor
Physician Executive MBA
College of Business Administration
The University of Tennessee
Knoxville, Tennessee
and
Senior Fellow
The Wharton School
The University of Pennsylvania
Philadelphia, Pennsylvania

AN ASPEN PUBLICATION®
Aspen Publishers, Inc.
Gaithersburg, Maryland
1999

This publication is designed to provide accurate and authoritative information in regard to the Subject Matter covered. It is sold with the understanding that the publisher is not engaged in rendering legal, accounting, or other professional service. If legal advice or other expert assistance is required, the service of a competent professional person should be sought. (From a Declaration of Principles jointly adopted by a Committee of the American Bar Association and a Committee of Publishers and Associations.)

Library of Congress Cataloging-in-Publication Data
The physician's essential MBA : what every physician leader needs to know / [edited by] Michael J. Stahl, Peter J. Dean.
p. cm.
Includes bibliographical references and index.
ISBN 0-8342-1244-7
1. Medicine—Practice—Management.   2. Physician executives—Education.   3. Physicians—Finance, Personal.   I. Stahl, Michael J.   II. Dean, Peter J., Ph.D.
[DNLM: 1. Practice Management, Medical—economics   2. Physician Executive–education.
W 80 P5773 1999]
R728.P495   1999
610′.68—dc21
DNLM/DLC
for Library of Congress   98-54872
CIP

About Aspen Publishers • For more than 35 years, Aspen has been a leading professional publisher in a variety of disciplines. Aspen's vast information resources are available in both print and electronic formats. We are committed to providing the highest quality information available in the most appropriate format for our customers. Visit Aspen's Internet site for more information resources, directories, articles, and a searchable version of Aspen's full catalog, including the most recent publications: **http://www.aspenpub.com**
Aspen Publishers, Inc. • The hallmark of quality in publishing
Member of the worldwide Wolters Kluwer group.

Editorial Services: Joan Sesma
Library of Congress Catalog Card Number: 98-54872
ISBN: 0-8342-1244-7

Printed in the United States of America
1   2   3   4   5

Table of Contents

About the Editors

Dr. Michael Stahl received his Ph.D. in Management from Rensselaer Polytechnic Institute. He is currently Director of the Physician Executive MBA Program and Distinguished Professor of Management in the College of Business Administration at The University of Tennessee, Knoxville. He teaches strategy in the Physician Executive MBA Program and in the full-time MBA program. Professional work experience includes program manager on the design and development of a communications satellite at the Space and Missile Systems Organization in Los Angeles, Head of the Management Department at Clemson University, and Associate Dean in the College of Business at UTK. Dr. Stahl has published over 50 journal articles in a variety of areas including Strategic Management and Total Quality Management and ten books including *Competing Globally Through Customer Value, Strategic Management: Total Quality and Global Competition,* and *Perspectives in Total Quality.* He is on the Board of Directors of the Florence Crittenton Agency and chairs that board's Development Committee.

Dr. Peter J. Dean received his Ph.D. at The University of Iowa and has taught there, as well as at Penn State and The University of Pennsylvania. Dr. Dean is a Senior Fellow at The Wharton School. He is an Associate Professor in the Physician Executive MBA Program at The University of Tennessee, Knoxville. His post-doctorate experience includes employment at Rockwell International Corporation in Iowa, and he has consulted for many companies including Johnson and Johnson, DuPont, Unisys, McNeil, and Microsoft. Dr. Dean has worked in Europe and Asia and lectured in Australia, Germany, Switzerland, India, Pakistan, and Sri Lanka. Courses taught include Business Ethics and Leadership, Managerial

Communication for Leaders, and Organizational Behavior and Change. He has published in many journals, edited and co-edited 5 books including *Performance Engineering at Work*, has been the editor for *Performance Improvement Quarterly* for 4 years, and received the 1993 Excellence in Teaching Award at Penn State University and the 1995 MBA Core Curriculum Cluster Teaching Award at The Wharton School.

About the Authors

Kate P. Atchley, MS. Ms. Atchley received her undergraduate degree in Psychology and her master's degree in Educational Administration from The University of Tennessee, Knoxville. In addition to her position with the College of Business Administration at The University of Tennessee, she has worked as an assessment and evaluation specialist in the department of Education and Training at the Tennessee Valley Authority. She also serves as a performance assessor for the Tennessee Assessment Center. She has consulted for various companies both nationally and in Bangkok, Thailand, including Shinawatra Company, Inc., The Management Development Center, The City of Oak Ridge, Lockheed-Martin Energy Systems, and BellSouth's L. M. Berry and Company. She has developed and conducted numerous workshops and training programs on conflict management, giving and receiving feedback, team building, and managing workplace diversity. Ms. Atchley is currently completing her requirements for a PhD in Industrial/Organizational Psychology at The University of Tennessee.

Bruce K. Behn, CPA, PhD. Dr. Behn joined the faculty after completing his doctorate at Arizona State University. He has an MBA from Arizona State University and a bachelor's degree from the University of Wisconsin-Madison. Prior to obtaining his PhD, Dr. Behn worked for Rockwell International in The Netherlands as the international financial coordinator, for Allen-Bradley Company as controller and financial analyst, and for KPMG Peat Marwick as senior auditor. He teaches statement analysis in the Taiwan and UT Executive MBA programs. He also teaches in various UT management development programs and in the business core of the Master of Accountancy program. Dr. Behn has been the recipient of a number of teaching and advising awards. He has also consulted with several companies including, most recently, the Knoxville Utility Board and Condor Freight Lines. Dr. Behn has published articles in the *Journal of Accounting Research, Contemporary Accounting Research, Advances in Accounting,* and the *Journal of Accountancy.*

Phillip R. Daves, PhD. Dr. Daves received his PhD in Business Administration (Finance) at the University of North Carolina at Chapel Hill. Currently, he is Associate Professor in the Department of Finance at The University of Tennessee. His research, teaching, and consulting interests are in asset valuation, derivative securities, firm valuation, and dividend policy. He has published academic research papers in such journals as *The Journal of Finance, Applied Financial Economics, The Financial Review,* and *The International Journal of Finance.* He has consulted in the areas of derivative securities and risk management education, business valuation, and acquisition analysis. Customers include First Tennessee National Bank; Dr. Caroll Coffee, DDS; University of Tennessee's Life Care Medical Associates, PA; IJ Corporation; Clayton Homes, Inc.; and Bush Brothers.

Sarah Fisher Gardial, PhD. Dr. Gardial is Associate Professor at The Department of Marketing, Logistics and Transportation. She earned her undergraduate and MBA degrees in Marketing from the University of Arkansas and her PhD in Marketing from The University of Houston. Her primary expertise and research interests are in the areas of customer value and customer satisfaction, the decision processes of customers and consumers, consumer information processing, and buyer-seller relationships. With Bob Woodruff, she is the co-author of *Know Your Customer: New Perspectives on Customer Value and Satisfaction.* This book is based on several years of research conducted in partnership with a variety of organizations. She has also written numerous articles for journal publications and conferences. Sarah has received several teaching awards over the years, is a frequent instructor in management development institutes at the UT College of Business Administration, and has conducted training and workshops for several organizations, including Procter and Gamble, Eastman Chemicals, and TRW.

Charles B. Garrison, PhD. Dr. Garrison received his PhD in Economics from The University of Kentucky and has been a member of the faculty at The University of Tennessee since 1967. His research and teaching interests are in the fields of macroeconomic theory, managerial economics. In 1989, he was the winner of the Outstanding MBA Faculty Award, and in 1995, he won the John B. Ross Award as the Outstanding Teacher in the College of Business Administration. He is the author of more than 25 articles in academic journals, has directed more than a dozen PhD theses, and has presented papers at a number of conferences in the United States and abroad. He has served as a consultant to the Organization for Economic Cooperation and Development, the Federal Deposit Insurance Corporation, and Oak Ridge National Laboratory.

Laura A. Gniatczyk, MS. Laura Gniatczyk earned her Bachelors in Business Administration from Adrian College in Michigan with a double major in Business and Psychology. She earned a master's in Industrial and Organizational Psychology from Illinois State University and is pursuing a PhD in the same discipline from the University of Tennessee. In addition to working with the Physician Executive MBA program, Laura currently works as a performance assessor and administrative coordinator for the Tennessee Assessment Center. Laura taught a senior level Personnel Management course and was a finalist for the College of Business Graduate Teaching Award. Further, Laura has consulted for a variety of companies, including Mitsubishi Motor Manufacture and Columbia/HCA. Laura also coordinated a grant project through the Central Illinois Private Industry Council to complete a multi-county workforce analysis to identify training needs for disadvantaged and recently unemployed workers.

Robert H. Jackson, Jr., MBA. Teaching statistics and computer science classes while completing his MBA, Mr. Jackson managed service software and support for Knoxville's two store ComputerLand franchise after graduation. Later hired by Martin Marietta Energy Systems (now Lockheed Martin), he co-designed and implemented an innovative in-house personal computer support center now supporting over 7,000 personal computers housed at the U.S. Department of Energy's national security facilities in Oak Ridge, Tennessee. Mr. Jackson founded Growth Technologies, Inc.—a diversified computer support services firm—and was its President and CEO until selling the firm to a consortium of its employees and investors in late 1993. Growth Technologies, Inc., provides computer database and data communication support for clients nationwide, including Dupont, the federal Environmental Protection Agency, Sears, and United Technologies corporations. Mr. Jackson continues in part-time technical consulting for a number of multinational firms. In his current role as Director of Administrative Systems for the University of Tennessee, Knoxville Division of Continuing Studies and Distance Education at the University of Tennessee at Knoxville, Mr. Jackson supervises the Telemedia, Marketing, and Information service units focusing on support of the University's outreach missions. Mr. Jackson also participates in technical and financial planning for the University of Tennessee's EdNet regional two–way video interactive education system and the Division of Continuing Studies Wide Area Network.

William Q. Judge, PhD. Dr. Judge received his PhD in Business Administration with a concentration in Strategic Management at The University of North Carolina at Chapel Hill. He is Associate Professor of Management at The University of Tennessee. Prior to entering academe, Dr. Judge was a strategic planning analyst for Armstrong World Industries in Pennsylvania. He currently serves as both Director and Policy and Strategy Committee Vice Chairman of St. Mary's Health System, Inc., in Knoxville. He is widely published and has received Outstanding Teaching awards.

Tom Ladd, PhD. Dr. Ladd is the Director of the Industrial and Organizational Psychology program and a professor in the Department of Management. He is a licensed psychologist and is founder and Director of the Tennessee Assessment Center. He attended Tennessee Technological University where he received both his Bachelor's and his Master's degree in Educational Psychology and Measurement. His doctorate, from the University of Georgia, is in Applied Psychology with a specialization in Industrial and Organizational Psychology. Dr. Ladd teaches undergraduate, MBA, and doctoral level courses in Personnel Administration, Employee Selection, Applied Psychology, Research Design, and Advanced Quantitative Methods. His research interests include employee selection, utility analysis and fair employment, manpower planning, and structural equation modeling. He has published numerous articles in scholarly journals and has held research grants from the National Science Foundation and the United States Air Force for the purpose of assessing utilities of personnel classification decisions.

Donald E. Lighter, MD. Dr. Lighter received his MD at St. Louis University and did a pediatric residency at The University of Illinois College of Medicine. Dr. Lighter later received a MBA from The University of Illinois. He joins the Physician Executive MBA team as an adjunct faculty member. He presently serves as Medical Director of First Mental Health Inc., as a consultant to the American Academy of Pediatrics, as an adjunct

Associate Professor for the Department of Pediatrics at Vanderbilt University Medical School, and as Clinical Associate Professor of Pediatrics at University of Tennessee's Medical Center, Knoxville Unit. He is involved in many health-related committees and community activities and has several publications on medical informatics and management.

Todd W. Little, BA. Todd Little earned his BA degree in Psychology from Clemson University with a minor in Business Administration. He is currently pursuing a PhD in Industrial/Organizational Psychology at The University of Tennessee. While at The University of Tennessee, Todd has been responsible for teaching several management courses with content ranging from organizational behavior to career planning. He has also served as a performance assessor for the Tennessee Assessment Center. In addition, Todd contracted with Tennessee Valley Authority (TVA) to evaluate their Total Quality Management program as well as the Quality Resources courses offered through TVA University. Prior to entering the doctoral program, Todd was employed by Private Healthcare Systems, Inc., and CapitalCare (an HMO subsidiary of Blue Cross Blue Shield of the National Capital Area).

Cheryl S. Massingale, JD, MBA. Dr. Massingale received her JD and MBA degrees from The University of Tennessee. She recently retired from her full-time faculty position as Associate Professor in the Department of Accounting and Business Law at the University of Tennessee and now joins the Physician Executive MBA team as an adjunct faculty member. During her twelve years at UT, she taught in the undergraduate and Master's of Accountancy Programs in the Management Development Center, and was a member of the MBA Core Faculty. She was selected as the MBA Outstanding Professor in 1997. She is past president of the Southeast Academy of Legal Studies in Business. Her research interests include healthcare and employment law, and she has published several articles for law reviews and legal journals and has presented numerous papers at conferences. She has served on the board of trustees for the Webb School of Knoxville, and Child and Family Services in Knoxville.

Curtis P. McLaughlin, DBA. Dr. McLaughlin has taught for 31 years at the schools of Business Administration and of Public Health at Harvard and the University of North Carolina at Chapel Hill. His current areas of interest are the delivery of quality services and the enhancement of services productivity in professional settings. He received degrees from Wesleyan University and Harvard University in chemistry, marketing, and operations management and has also managed in industry and consulted extensively. Dr. McLaughlin is the author of over 200 publications, many of which deal with the development of quality improvement programs in health care, with product line management in mental health, and with the organization of care units to provide appropriate focus and coverage in health services. He just completed co-authoring a book on managed care, privatization, and public health for Aspen Publishers. His recent research has appeared in *Medical Care, New England Journal of Medicine, Management Science, International Journal Of Service Industry Management, Health Care Management Review,* and *Joint Commission Journal on Quality Improvement.* He is on the editorial boards of *Health Care Management Review, Journal of Services Research,* and *International Journal of Service Industry Management.*

Charles Noon, PhD. Dr. Noon received his PhD in Industrial & Operations Engineering from The University of Michigan. He is now Associate Professor of Management Science at the University of Tennessee. Dr. Noon's research and teaching interests include operations management and logistics modeling. His papers in these areas have appeared in *Operations Research, European Journal of Operational Research, INFOR,* and the *Journal of the Operational Research Society.* His recent projects involve the development of GIS-based decision support systems for the Tennessee Valley Authority, Lockheed-Martin Energy Systems, and the Electric Power Research Institute. In addition, he is co-developer of a one-week UT management development program entitled, "GIS for Business and Logistics." Dr. Noon was selected as a Stokely Scholar (1995–97) of The University of Tennessee College of Business Administration and was the recipient of the 1992 Outstanding Young Engineer Award from his alma mater, the University of Louisville.

Amy W. Ray, PhD. Dr. Ray received her PhD in Business with a concentration in Accounting and Information Systems at Virginia Polytechnic Institute and State University. She is now Associate Professor in the Department of Accounting and Business Law at the University of Tennessee. Dr. Ray's teaching experience includes Electronic Commerce, Object-Oriented Analysis and Design, Expert Systems, Network Security, and Accounting Information Systems. Most of her research involves management of information technology and she is widely published in many journals including the *Journal of Management Information Systems, Information and Management, Journal of Information Systems,* and *Journal of*

Strategic Information Systems. During the current 1998–1999 academic year she is serving as Chair-Elect of the Information Systems Section of the American Accounting Association and is a member of the AAA/ AICPA Technology Visioning Task Force and also the AAA/AICPA Technology Toolkit Project Team. As part of Arthur Andersen's Faculty Residency Program, she spent several months during 1998 working with AA's Global Best Practices and Virtual Learning Network groups.

David L. Sylwester, PhD. Dr. Sylwester received his PhD in statistics from Stanford University. He is a Professor in the Department of Statistics in the College of Business Administration at The University of Tennessee. Dr. Sylwester previously worked at The University of Vermont in the departments of Mathematics, and Epidemiology & Community Health. At UT, he is involved in developing and teaching courses through the college's Management Development Center. Dr. Sylwester is active in the American Statistical Association and currently serves on the board of directors as Treasurer of the Association. He is widely published primarily on the topics of Biostatistics and statistical process control.

Preface

The health care industry is one of the most dramatically changing industries in the United States at the dawn of the new millenium. There are changes in strategy, demand for health care, government's role, organizational structures, customers, disease management, financing, outcomes measurement, health care operations, leadership, law, ethics, quality, and information systems. These changes are occurring so rapidly, that today's provider can no longer sit back and continue to deliver medicine as in the past, partly because the financial risk has shifted to providers.

Few environmental changes have had the impact on the health care industry in the United States as the growth in health care expenditures. Over the last two decades, the health care industry has seen robust growth measured both in absolute dollars, about $1 trillion, and as a percentage of the total domestic economy, about 14%. As the population ages and demands more health care services, and as the political system extends health care services to more, many forecast that the growth in health care expenditures will continue for the foreseeable future both in terms of the percent of the total domestic economy and absolute dollars.

One of the market-based approaches to control those costs has been the rapid growth in managed care. As a measure of that growth in managed care, the number of members enrolled in health maintenance organizations (HMOs) has exploded in the last few years. *Business Week* (June 15, 1998) estimated that about 90 million members were enrolled in HMOs in mid 1998. HMOs have grown in popularity primarily because they charge significantly less in monthly premiums than traditional medical insurance based on the traditional fee–for–service approach.

HMOs usually use designated physicians (primary care physicians—PCPs) as gatekeepers, pre-approved lists of providers, and pre-approved list of pharmaceuticals. Thus, HMOs control health care expenditures in part by controlling the utilization of pre-selected providers and pharmaceutical products. HMOs also negotiate discounted fees for the services they purchase from the pre-selected providers, or the HMOs provide capitated payments to physicians. Thus, many physicians have seen their autonomy to practice medicine and their incomes from clinical practice at risk.

One measure of the breadth of change in the health care industry comes from a 1997 environmental assessment performed by Deloitte & Touche for the millenium. Deloitte & Touche summarized eight big trends in the health care industry for the millenium. One of the trends, "New Roles for Physicians," is of particular interest to this book. In January 1998, we conducted a survey in class among the 24 physicians from 11 different states enrolled in the Physician Executive MBA (PEMBA) at The University of Tennessee. All 24 physicians agreed with the trend: "Physicians' roles will become increasingly important in health care management and government health care policy-making."

If 100% of the physicians in PEMBA in 1998 and Deloitte & Touche in 1997 were correct, then we have an answer to one of the questions posed by this book: "Why should a physician pursue an MBA?" If physicians assume increasingly important roles as health care executives, then physician leaders need to acquire the knowledge and skills to fulfill those executive roles. Pursuing an MBA focused on physician leadership is one way to acquire the knowledge and skills.

An April 1996 *USA Today* survey indicated that 38% of the 700,000 USA physicians either had or were planning on getting an MBA. Thus, there appears to be a large market for physician focused MBAs. Therefore, this book has at least three purposes.

- Help physicians decide about getting an MBA.
- Give physicians a preview of MBA content.
- Help spouses understand why their favorite physician is getting an MBA and what the physician will learn.

If this book accomplishes those purposes, then it will have been successful and added to the growing knowledge base on physician leadership.

Michael J. Stahl and Peter J. Dean

Acknowledgements

As co-editors, we would like to acknowledge the work of so many others that made this book become a reality. Without that team effort, this book would still be only a concept.

First, we recognize the author team. These 17 professionals designed, drafted, and re-drafted the book's integrative material in near record time. We are proud to call them colleagues.

Charles B. Garrison
Curtis P. McLaughlin
Sarah F. Gardial
Bruce K. Behn
Phillip R. Daves
Charles Noon
Donald E. Lighter
William Q. Judge
Kate Atchley
Laura Gniatczyk
Tom Ladd
Todd Little
Cheryl S. Massingale
David L. Sylwester
Donald E. Lighter
Amy W. Ray
Robert H. Jackson, Jr.

We also recognize the work of Mr. Thomas Brown, Program Coordinator, Physician Executive MBA, University of Tennessee. Tom developed and maintained web pages with the draft chapters so that the co-editors and the author team could read all the chapters and insure consistency.

Certainly, we must acknowledge the help of Ms. Sandy Cannon, Acquisition Editor at Aspen. Sandy guided our book proposal through the approval process at Aspen and established a process to bring the book to market in near record time.

PART I

Change and Strategy in the Health Care Industry

CHAPTER 1

Strategy in the Mutating Health Care Industry: Strategic Planning Processes for Changes in Managed Care

Michael J. Stahl

TABLE OF CONTENTS

EXECUTIVE SUMMARY

The health care industry is one of the most dramatically changing industries in the United States at the dawn of the new millenium. There are changes in demographics, medical technology, the role of the government, delivery, organizational structures, economics, and, certainly, financing. These sea changes are occurring so rapidly that today's provider can no longer sit back and continue to deliver medicine as he or she did in the past. Many sectors of the industry, ranging from physicians through hospitals, pharmaceutical companies, and other suppliers have realized that they must analyze these changes and develop new strategies to deal with them in order to grow and prosper.

This chapter discusses strategy, stages of managed care, and a strategic planning process to deal with these changes in the United States health care industry. Hopefully, by acquiring the skills and knowledge concerning such business issues, physician leaders will be able to proactively plan for some of the changes and implement new strategies rather than passively react to strategies formulated by others.

STRATEGIC ENVIRONMENTAL ANALYSIS

In the rapidly changing health care industry, the failure to understand the new environment and adapt may lead to demise. Just as the study of biology tells us that organisms must adapt over time to survive in new environments, organizational science tells us that organizations adapt to new environments. However, because of business competition and government influence, organizations must adapt much more quickly than biological organisms. To design a strategy, we need to understand the features of the environment external to the organization

The Strategic Management Process

The strategic management process involves the range of strategic decisions from planning the strategy to the control of operations. There are three major steps in the strategic management process: strategy formulation, implementation, and evaluation and control. *Strategy formulation* involves the decisions that determine the organization's mission, vision and values, and establishes the organization's objectives and strategies. Some refer to strategy formulation as strategic planning. *Strategy implementa-*

tion involves the activities and decisions that are made to install the strategic plan. Some refer to strategy implementation as operational management. *Strategic evaluation and control* involves the activities and decisions that keep the process on track. Evaluation and control include following up on goal accomplishment and feeding back the results to decision makers. Figure 1–1 depicts these three major steps of strategy formulation, implementation, and evaluation and control in the strategic management process.

Throughout recorded history, there have been various managerial and organizational practices in vogue to fit the demands of the times. Leaders must change strategies and managerial practices to fit the environment if they wish their organizations to survive and prosper. To effectively formulate strategy, strategic decision makers need to understand and forecast environmental trends.

Internal Strengths and Weaknesses and External Opportunities and Threats (SWOT) Analysis

To understand environmental trends, managers must analyze conditions in the internal environment of the organization *and* conditions in the external environment (Stahl & Grigsby, 1997). This analysis of the internal environment and the external environment is so pervasive in strategic planning that it has its own acronym. This analysis of internal Strengths and Weaknesses and external Opportunities and Threats is called a *SWOT Analysis*. Exhibit 1–1 shows the primary internal and external issues examined in a SWOT Analysis.

Conditions internal to the organization are called *internal strengths and weaknesses*. A *strength* is a condition or issue internal to the organization that may lead to a customer benefit or a competitive advantage. Alternatively, a *weakness* is a condition or issue internal to the organization that may lead to negative customer value or a competitive disadvantage. Most of these internal strengths and weaknesses are the result of prior management decisions.

Internal strengths and weaknesses are inside the organization and under the influence of managers. Therefore, it is assumed that the weaknesses can be changed. External threats can be more trying than the internal conditions because external threats are not under the control of the firm's managers.

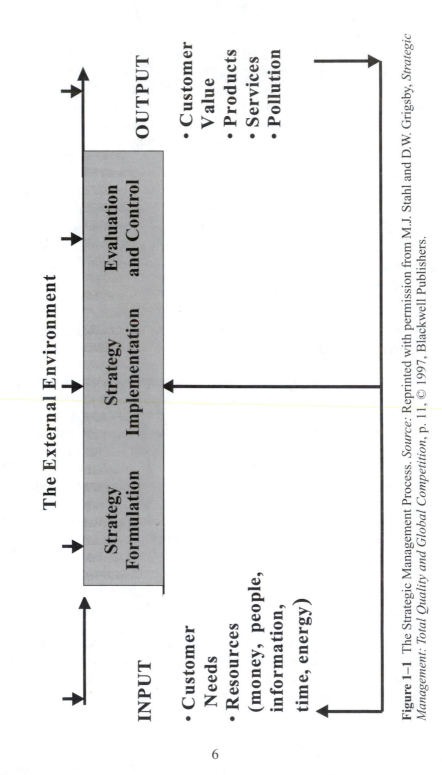

The External Environment

INPUT

- **Customer Needs**
- **Resources (money, people, information, time, energy)**

Strategy Formulation

Strategy Implementation

Evaluation and Control

OUTPUT

- **Customer Value**
- **Products**
- **Services**
- **Pollution**

Figure 1–1 The Strategic Management Process. *Source:* Reprinted with permission from M.J. Stahl and D.W. Grigsby, *Strategic Management: Total Quality and Global Competition*, p. 11, © 1997, Blackwell Publishers.

Exhibit 1–1 Primary SWOT Issues

INTERNAL STRENGTHS AND WEAKNESSES
- Horizontal systems and processes
- Organizational structure
- Corporate culture
- Management
- Financial position
- Operations
- Marketing
- Human resources
- Research and development
- Information systems

EXTERNAL OPPORTUNITIES AND THREATS
- Customer value trends
- Social trends
- Demographic trends
- Economic trends
- Technological trends
- Regulatory trends
- Physical trends
- Competitive trends

Source: Reprinted with permission from M.J. Stahl and D.W. Grigsby, *Strategic Management: Total Quality and Global Competition*, p. 30, © 1997, Blackwell Publishers.

An *opportunity* is an issue or condition in the environment external to the firm that may help it reach its goals. A *threat* is an issue or condition in the external environment that may prevent the firm from reaching its goals. Very strong external opportunities or threats may even cause the firm to evolve its goals and strategies.

Opportunities and threats in the external environment are not under the direct control of the firm's managers. However, external opportunities and threats must be responded to if the firm wishes to remain healthy and grow. Analyzing the external environment is labeled as *environmental scanning*. High organizational performance is associated with the frequency and breadth of environmental scanning (Daft, Sormunen, & Parks, 1988).

The trends listed in Exhibit 1–1 under External Opportunities and Threats may be opportunities or may be threats, depending on the nature of the trend. Unlike the issues listed under Internal Strengths and Weaknesses, external trends are not under the control of management. However, management can anticipate and respond to the external trends with adequate environmental scanning and strategic planning.

Economic and Financing Changes

Few environmental changes have had the impact on the health care industry in the United States as has the growth in health care expenditures. Over the last two decades, the health care industry has seen robust growth measured both in absolute dollars, about $1 trillion, and as a percentage of the total domestic economy, about 14%. As the population ages and demands more health care services, and as medical technology becomes more complex, many people in the industry forecast that the growth will continue for the foreseeable future. Figure 1–2 shows the historical and forecasted growth in health care expenditures both in absolute dollars and as a percentage of the total domestic economy.

The financing of that growth by the Federal Government has produced many changes in the practice of medicine in this country. The Federal Government has become the largest third-party payer in this country with the Health Care Financing Administration to administer its programs to providers. Figure 1–3 depicts the growth in Federal Government expenditures and the relative decline in private expenditures.

Eight Big Health Care Trends for the Millenium

One measure of the breadth of change in the health care industry comes from an Environmental Assessment performed by Deloitte & Touche (1997) for the millenium. Exhibit 1–2 summarizes eight big trends in the health care industry for the Millenium forecasted by Deloitte & Touche. The first trend, "Managed Care Marches On," and the sixth trend, "New Roles for Physicians," are of particular interest to our study of strategy in the health care industry.

The growth of Managed Care has been having such a pervasive role in the entire health care industry that the next section is devoted to the topic. To summarize, the authors of the report expect even greater enrollment in managed care plans with resultant changes among physicians, hospitals,

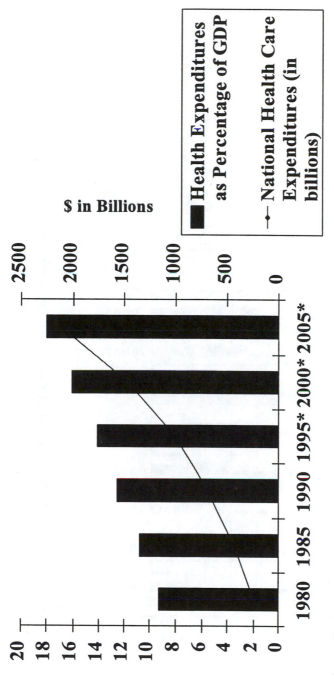

Figure 1–2 Growth in National Health Care Expenditures in Dollars and as a Percentage of Gross Domestic Product. *Source:* Reprinted from Congressional Budget Office, 1996.

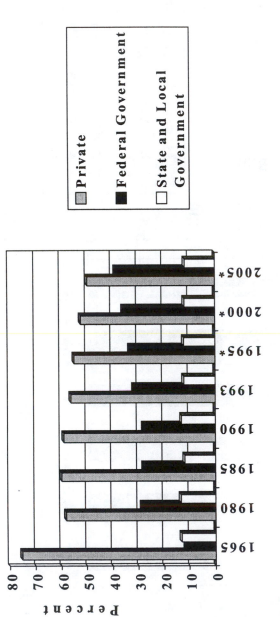

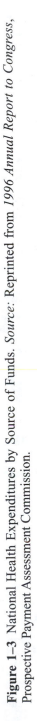

*Projected

Figure 1–3 National Health Expenditures by Source of Funds. *Source:* Reprinted from *1996 Annual Report to Congress,* Prospective Payment Assessment Commission.

Exhibit 1–2 Eight Big Health Care Trends

1. Managed Care Marches On
2. Changing Government Roles
3. Cost Reduction
4. Consolidation
5. Consumer Involvement
6. New Roles For Physicians
7. Defining and Demonstrating Quality
8. Information Technology

Source: Data from 1997 Environmental Assessment, *Redesigning Health Care for the Millennium: An Assessment of the Health Care Environment in the United States*, pp. 109–112, © 1997, VHA, Inc. and Deloitte & Touche, LLP.

pharmaceutical companies, other suppliers, and whole new networks among providers in the new era of managed care.

In January 1998, we conducted a survey in a class among the 24 physicians from 11 different states enrolled in the Physician Executive MBA (PEMBA) at The University of Tennessee. All 24 physicians agreed with the trend concerning "New Roles for Physicians." Specifically, 100% of the physicians agreed with the statement "Physicians' roles will become increasingly important in health care management and government health care policy-making" (VHA, Inc. and Deloitte & Touche, 1997).

If 100% of the physicians in PEMBA in 1998 and Deloitte & Touche in 1997 were correct, then we have an answer to one of the questions posed by this book: "Why should an MD pursue an MBA?" If physicians assume increasingly important roles as health care executives, then physician leaders need to acquire the knowledge and skills to fulfill those executive roles. Pursuing an MBA focused on physician leadership is one way to acquire the knowledge and skills.

MANAGED CARE

What does even greater enrollments in managed care plans portend? Will there be continued cost pressures? Will those cost pressures impact the income and the very employability of physicians? Will providers assume some of the risk for revenues? Will third-party payers increasingly control the interactions among physicians and patients? The growth of managed care has had such profound changes in the conduct of the entire health care industry that we need to examine that growth to gain some insight into the questions.

Health Maintenance Organization (HMO) Growth

One of the best measures of the stage of managed care is the number of members enrolled in Health Maintenance Organizations (HMOs). *Business Week* (*The healer's revenge* 1998) recently estimated that about 90 million members were enrolled in HMOs in mid-1998. HMOs have grown in popularity primarily because they charge significantly less in monthly premiums than traditional medical insurance based on the traditional fee–for–service approach.

HMOs usually use designated physicians (primary care physicians) as gatekeepers, preapproved lists of providers, and preapproved lists of pharmaceuticals. Thus, HMOs control health care expenditures in at least two ways. First, HMOs control the utilization of preselected providers and pharmaceutical products. Second, HMOs negotiate discounted fees for the services they purchase from the preselected providers, or the HMOs provide capitated payments to physicians. "Capitation is a set amount of money received or paid out; it is based on membership rather than on services delivered and usually is expressed in units of PMPM (Per Member Per Month)" (Kongstvedt, 1996).

Many changes have been occurring in the health care industry, which are compliments of the cost pressures from HMOs. One noteworthy change is that in an attempt to control costly hospital stays, ambulatory care has become very popular (Melville, 1993). An allied change associated with attempts to control health care expenditures has been the dramatic decline in the typical number of inpatient days. Whereas the number of inpatient days per 1,000 population was a little over 1,200 in 1980, the Advisory Board has recently estimated that the number of inpatient days per 1,000 population will be less than 200 in the near future, for a decline of over 80% (Capitation Strategies, 1994).

Between 1994 and 1997, the profitability of HMOs declined dramatically. During that time period, their average profit margins declined from 2.4% to minus 1.2% (HMO profitability, 1998). Such profit declines, coupled with increased popularity, indicate that HMOs will continue to exert substantial cost pressures on providers.

Oversupply of Physicians

Just as managed care has been associated with decreased utilization of hospital facilities, managed care has been associated with decreased utilization of physicians in attempts to control costs. Because HMOs are particularly interested in controlling the utilization of specialists, oversupply is worse among specialists. The *Dartmouth Atlas of Health Care* (1996) recently estimated that all specialists are oversupplied by about 80%.

Partly for this oversupply condition, the percentage of self-employed physicians has dropped from 80% to 55% over the past 10 years (Physician Compensation, 1997). Record numbers of physicians have been selling their practices to management companies or hospitals, joining group practices without walls, joining Management Services Organizations, merging their practices, or joining Physician Hospital Organizations.

Multiple Stages of Managed Care

Providers in the health care industry need to thoroughly understand a force as powerful as managed care so they can survive and provide the kind of patient care they deem appropriate and their patients demand. Two of the better models of managed care recognize that managed care has advanced at different rates in different cities and regions. Coile (1997) did a fine job analyzing four stages of managed care with up to 40% HMO Penetration. Shortell, Gillies, Anderson, Erickson, and Mitchell (1996) did a fine job analyzing two stages of managed care between 40% and 100% HMO Penetration. Exhibit 1–3 summarizes those stages of managed care. Income to physicians and profit margins to health care provider organizations often decline dramatically through the first few stages of managed care. The role of providers often changes from providing the best possible health care at any cost to providing health care at an affordable cost. The change in financing from fee-for-service to capitated payments reinforces new behavior and new organizational forms.

Each stage of managed care has its own characteristics, strategies and organization types for providers, HMOs, and insurers. Analyzing each is beyond the scope of this chapter. However, an MBA program for physician leaders should analyze managed care in much greater depth than here with particular emphasis on appropriate strategies for various stages of managed care.

Exhibit 1–3 Multiple Stages of Managed Care

Stage	HMO Penetration	Stage Title
1	<5%	Can't Spell HMO
2	5–15%	Managed Care Gets Aggressive
3	15–25%	Managed Care Penetration
4	25–40%	Managed Competition
C	40–60%	Consolidated "Advanced Cost" Market
D	>60%	Strict Managed Care "Value" Market

Source: Data from R.C. Coile, *The Five Stages of Managed Care: Strategies for Providers, HMOs, and Suppliers,* © 1997, American College of Healthcare Executives and S. Shortell et al., *Remaking Health Care in America,* © 1996, Jossey-Bass.

THE STRATEGIC PLAN

After the SWOT Analysis has been performed with the analysis of internal strengths and weaknesses, as well as external opportunities and threats including stage of managed care, then physician leaders are able to formulate the strategic plan. Physician leaders can use the process of strategic planning to educate other providers in the organization about the changes in the health care environment and the impact of managed care. Then, physician leaders can lead their organization and their colleagues into the future and make decisions appropriate for the new managed care environment. Indeed, a prime purpose of developing a strategic plan is to have a guide for making strategic decisions.

The *strategic plan* includes a mission, vision, values, objectives, and strategies. Figure 1–4 summarizes those elements. Some plans may combine some of the five elements into three or four elements. For the sake of analysis, we will explore all five elements.

The strategic plan should be formulated to capitalize on external opportunities and internal strengths, and to work around external threats and internal weaknesses. *Grow-and-invest situations* are those in which firms can capitalize on external opportunities with internal strengths. For example, in the era of managed care, a hospital and physicians may find that an outpatient surgery center is a way to grow. *Shrinkage or withdrawal situations* are those in which firms have significant internal weaknesses or external threats that they cannot overcome. In an era of managed care and

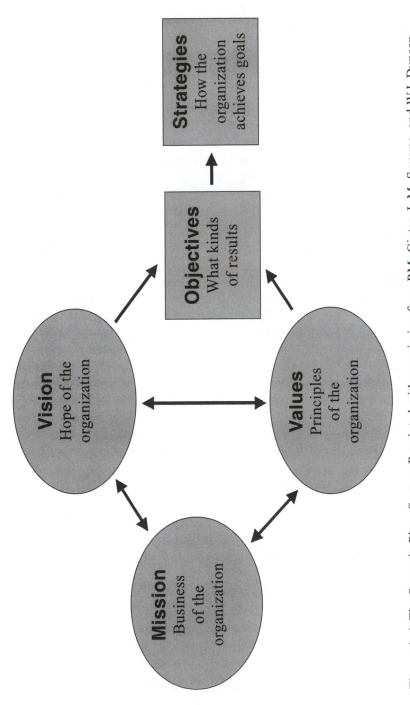

Figure 1–4 The Strategic Plan. *Source:* Reprinted with permission from P.M. Ginter, L.M. Swayne, and W.J. Duncan, *Strategic Management of Health Care Organizations*, p. 141, © 1998, Blackwell Publishers.

capitated payments, a provider organization may withdraw from seeing HMO patients because the payment stream is too low for the providers' cost structure.

Mission

A *mission statement* describes what business(es) the organization is in. The mission indicates why the organization exists. Although the mission refers to the whole enterprise, there is only one mission statement per enterprise.

The mission statement should be written from the perspective of the customers rather than the stockholders, owners, employees, or any other group. Mission statements usually describe the organization's chief products or services, the target customers or markets served, the geographical domain, the customer value provided, and the organization's key activities and functions. An example of a mission statement printed in Eli Lilly's Annual Report (1991) follows: "Eli Lilly and Company is a global research-based corporation that develops, manufactures, and markets pharmaceuticals, medical instruments and diagnostic products, and animal health products. The company markets its products in 110 countries around the world." A primary function of Lilly's management is understanding what the customers in 110 countries require.

Vision

A *vision statement* is a future-oriented statement of what the organization aspires to be. A vision statement is meant to be future oriented, challenging and inspirational, and it is meant to empower employees and customers, and provide guidance.

An example of a vision statement is from the OrNda Health Corporation (1992), one of the largest for-profit hospital organizations in the United States: "OrNda Health Corp will be recognized for creativity and excellence in delivering value-added hospital and related services that meet or exceed patient, physician, and payor expectations."

Values

Values are the principles guiding an organization. These principles may make the organization unique. Values often relate to ethical behavior and socially responsible decision making. (*See* Chapter 12.)

An example of a statement of values comes from the Cleveland Clinic Foundation (1994): "The Cleveland Clinic Foundation was established by visionary leaders who believed in simple, guiding principles. Five fundamental values form the foundation of the Cleveland Clinic culture: Collaboration, Quality, Integrity, Compassion and Commitment."

Objectives

After the *why* of the business has been defined, it is appropriate to describe the *what*. *Objectives or goals* refer to the kinds of results the organization seeks to achieve. Corporate objectives or goals refer to results targeted for the entire corporation. Goals can also exist at the business level, the functional-area level (like marketing), and lower levels in the organization.

Objectives should be specific, measurable, time phased, and realistic. The realistic characteristic explains why objectives are considered *after* the mission and vision. The mission and vision statements broadly determine what is achievable and desirable, as well as the context. For example, a 30% annual rate of growth in sales may be realistic for a rapidly growing biotechnology company like Amgen. However, such an objective is not realistic for a local hospital in a stable market. Increasing attention is being paid to market share and sales growth objectives as these goals show relative changes in value realized by customers. One year or less refers to a short-term objective, and five years or more refer to a long-term objective. The time between refers to a medium-term objective.

There are three themes that may be found in objectives. One is growth. In a *growth* theme, the organization attempts to grow and expand through significantly increased sales. Many biotechnology companies and outpatient services companies pursue growth. Another theme is *stability*. Organizations in mature environments, like medical supplies, that do not expect significant growth pursue stability. The third theme is *restructuring*. Restructuring refers to a series of actions aimed at downsizing or cutting back the scope of the organization. In the early stages of managed care, many hospitals have restructured the organization to deal with intense cost pressures. (*See* Chapter 4.)

Strategies

After the objectives have been decided, the leaders can decide how to achieve them. *Strategy* refers to *how* the organization will achieve its objectives. The choice of strategies at the corporate, business, and functional levels is central to the understanding of strategic management.

Henry Mintzberg (1978) described strategy *as* "a pattern in a stream of decisions." He portrayed this idea by describing the patterns in the many decisions made at Volkswagenwerk over a 54-year period. From those decisions and the patterns in the decisions, the company's strategy of low priced transportation may be spotted throughout the years that the Volkswagen was marketed throughout the world.

Mintzberg's idea that strategy is "a pattern in a stream of decisions" has two important implications. First, strategy is not necessarily apparent from the analysis of just one decision. To fully understand strategy, it must be viewed in the context of several decisions and the consistency among the decisions. Second, the organization must be aware of decision alternatives in all of its decisions. Strategy may be viewed as the logic that governs the firm's choices among all its decision options.

Is strategy always a purposeful process? Is strategy always the outcome of a planned effort toward goals that results in a pattern in a series of decisions? Might strategy also be the result of leaders simply "muddling through" without an explicit plan? The cumulative effect of making small decisions regularly can result in a pattern in the stream of decisions.

Mintzberg and Waters (1985) contrasted *deliberate strategy* with *emergent strategy*. Deliberate strategy had been viewed as a result of the strategic planning process. Deliberate strategy consists of an organization deciding on its goals and implementing intended strategy to realize the goals. This view of strategy as a deliberate process neglects several possibilities (Mintzberg, 1990). Sometimes an organization may not intentionally set strategy. The organization's strategy may emerge from the lower levels of the organization because of its daily activities. Such emergent strategies might also be the result of the implementation process. Alterations in goals based on feedback during implementation may produce strategies that vary from their original design. *Emergent strategies* are those strategies actually in place in the organization.

QUO VADIS?

The concept that emergent strategies may be different from deliberate strategies is especially relevant to strategic evaluation and control in the health care industry today. Given the changes that are being wrought by the forces of managed care, many physician leaders and health care organizations will try new strategies, new organizational alliances, and new structures. Some of those innovations will work and some will go awry. Physician leaders need to understand the changes in the health care industry environment, especially changes in managed care, to develop a successful strategy and to lead their organizations and colleagues in the future. To effect that strategic leadership, physician leaders need far more knowledge and skills of such business issues than they ever learned in medical school. How will you lead change and develop strategy in your organization?

GLOSSARY

capitation. a set amount of money received or paid out; it is based on membership rather than on services delivered, and it usually is expressed in units of PMPM (Per Member Per Month).

deliberate strategy. consists of an organization deciding on its goals and implementing intended strategy to realize the goals.

emergent strategies. those strategies actually in place in the organization.

environmental scanning. analyzing the external environment.

grow-and-invest situations. those in which firms can capitalize on external opportunities with internal strengths.

mission statement. describes what business(es) the organization is in.

objectives or **goals.** refer to the kinds of results the organization seeks to achieve.

opportunity. an issue or condition in the environment external to the firm that may help it reach its goals.

restructuring. refers to a series of actions aimed at downsizing or cutting back the scope of the organization.

shrinkage or **withdrawal situations.** those in which firms have significant internal weaknesses or external threats that they cannot overcome.

strategic evaluation and control. involves the activities and decisions that keep the process on track.

strategic plan. includes a mission, vision, values, objectives, and strategies.

strategy. refers to how the organization will achieve its objectives; **strategy.** a pattern in a stream of decisions.

strategy formulation. involves the decisions that determine the organization's mission, vision, and values, and establishes the organization's objectives and strategies.

strategy implementation. involves the activities and decisions that are made to install the strategic plan.

strength. a condition or issue internal to the organization that may lead to a customer benefit or a competitive advantage.

SWOT Analysis. an analysis of internal Strengths and Weaknesses and external Opportunities and Threats.

threat. an issue or condition in the external environment that may prevent the firm from reaching its goals.

values. the principles guiding an organization.

vision statement. a future-oriented statement of what the organization aspires to be.

weakness. a condition or issue internal to the organization that may lead to negative customer value or a competitive disadvantage.

REFERENCES

Capitation strategies. (1994). Washington, DC: Advisory Board Company.

Coile, R. C. (1997). *The five stages of managed care: Strategies for providers, HMOs, and suppliers.* Chicago: American College of Healthcare Executives.

Daft, R. L., Sormunen, J., & Parks, D. (1988, March–April). Chief executive scanning, environmental characteristics, and company performance. *Strategic Management Journal, 9,* 123–139.

Dartmouth Medical School. (1996). *Dartmouth atlas of health care.* Hanover, NH: Author.

Eli Lilly & Co. (1991). *Report to shareholders.* Indianapolis, IN: Author.

HMO profitability. (1998, June). *On Managed Care, 3,* 1.

Kongstvedt, P. (1996). *The managed health care handbook* (3rd ed.). Gaithersburg, MD: Aspen Publishers.

Melville, B. (1993). Ambulatory care site: A vital strategic decision. *Health Care Competition Week, 10,* 1–4.

Mintzberg, H. (1978). Patterns in strategy formation. *Management Science, 24,* 934–948.

Mintzberg, H. (1990, March–April). The design school. *Strategic Management Journal, 11,* 171–196.

Mintzberg, H., & Waters, J. A. (1985). Of strategies, deliberate and emergent. *Strategic Management Journal, 6,* 257–271.

OrNda Health Corp. (1992). *A new force in health care: Annual report.* Nashville, TN: Author.

Physician compensation: What doctors want. (1997). *Journal of Medical Practice Management, 57,* 17–18.

Shortell, S., Gillies, R., Anderson, D., Erickson, K., & Mitchell, J. (1996). *Remaking health care in America.* San Francisco: Jossey-Bass, Publishers.

Stahl, M. J., & Grigsby, D. W. (1997). *Strategic management.* Oxford, England: Blackwell Publishers.

The Cleveland Clinic Foundation. (1994). *Division of health affairs: Annual report.* Cleveland, OH: Author.

The healers' revenge: Doctors and hospitals begin to wrest control from HMOs. (1998, June 15). *Business Week,* p. 70.

VHA, Inc. and Deloitte & Touche (1997). Environmental assessment. In *Redesigning health care for the millenium: An assessment of the health care environment in the United States* (p. 111). Irving, TX: VHA, Inc. and Detroit, MI: Deloitte & Touche LLP.

CHAPTER 2

Economics Of Health Care Policy

Charles B. Garrison

TABLE OF CONTENTS

EXECUTIVE SUMMARY

Physician leaders are vitally concerned with the long-term viability of the Medicare and Medicaid programs. The ability of these programs to survive and thrive depends on the ability of the working-age population to support payments to future recipients. This chapter addresses the prospects for long-run growth of income per capita in the United States and for long-run behavior of the ratio of working-age population to retirement-age population. A model of long-run economic growth, the augmented Solow model, is used to explore the likelihood that improvements in income per worker will offset the predicted decline in the ratio of working-age population to retirement-age population. According to the augmented Solow model, continued improvements in economy wide technology, a high national saving rate, increases in human capital, and the avoidance of severe recessions are necessary to achieve such an outcome.

The challenge to the ability of the economy to support Social Security and the two medical care programs will be especially acute during the period 2010–2030. During that period, the percent of the United States population accounted for by the 65-and-over age group will increase from 13.2% to 20.0%, compared to 12.7% in 1996. Consequently, the decline in the working-age population to retirement-age population ratio also will be most pronounced during the period after 2010. Maintaining a high national saving rate from now until the year 2030 will be crucial to supporting those programs. A high national saving rate permits the economy to devote more of its output to investment in new physical capital, including machinery and equipment, which raise output per worker. National saving includes not only personal saving but also business saving and government saving. Government saving is positive if a government budget surplus is achieved but it is negative if a deficit occurs. A critical element in maintaining high national saving is for the federal government to avoid a return to the era of large budget deficits.

TRENDS AND PROJECTIONS

Medical care is an economic good just as food, clothing, housing, and entertainment are economic goods. The purpose of medical care is to improve the stock of health of people. It is health, not medical care itself, which brings utility to the consumer of medical care. Thus we may think of an individual's stock of health as an increasing function of the quantity of medical care consumed. As with other goods, production of health by means of medical care implies that resources (physical capital and labor) must be used, and this implies that these resources are not available to produce alternative goods and services. An increase in the production of medical care, given the quantity of resources and the level of technology, requires that society give up some amount of other goods, called X. This important concept is illustrated in Figure 2–1.

Medical care differs from other goods and services, however, in some important respects. In particular, the following characteristics are more important than for most other goods and services: the extent of government intervention, the importance of insurance as a payment system, asymmetric information, and uncertainty of medical outcomes. In this chapter we are especially interested in government intervention as a crucial element in the delivery of medical care and in providing insurance. Government health care policy is especially important in providing medical insurance for the elderly and low-income population in the form of the Medicare and Medicaid programs.

Demographic and economic trends create a great deal of concern among physician leaders and policy makers regarding the future of the Medicare and Medicaid programs. The Social Security disability and survivors' programs are subject to the same concern. The concern revolves

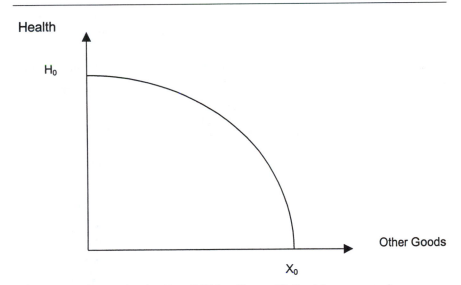

Figure 2–1 The Production Possibilities Curve. If all of the economy's resources were devoted to the production of health, the amount of health produced would be H_0, and the amount of other goods produced would be zero. Moving downward, the slope of the curve shows the amount of health that must be forgone as the production of X is increased by one unit. A movement upward along the curve shows the amount of other goods that must be sacrificed to produce one more unit of health.

around the long-run (20 to 50 years) projection that the ratio of the number of workers to the number of retirees and others eligible to receive benefits will decline. That is, the projection that the ratio will decline induces fears that all three of the programs will encounter serious financial difficulties in the future, and that overcoming the decline in the ratio will require onerous tax increases on the working population in the future.

The aging of the United States population is the chief concern with regard to the impact of long-term trends on the ability of the society to support the Medicare, Medicaid, and Social Security programs. The aging trend is not new: the median age of the population, after falling from 30.2 years in 1950 to 28.0 years in 1970, has risen steadily since 1970. It is projected to continue to rise through the first quarter of the 21st century, reaching 38.0 by 2025 (see Table 2–1). There are two reasons for the concern with aging: (1) The stock of health of an individual declines with age, and therefore the elderly tend to use more medical care than the younger population; (2) an increase in the fraction of the population that is retired tends to reduce the ratio of people who are working (and consequently contributing to the Social Security and Medicare programs) to the people who are retired and receiving benefits from the programs. We term this ratio the "support ratio."

Table 2–2 shows support ratios for the United States, Japan, and the United Kingdom. The long-term trend clearly is downward for each coun-

Table 2–1 The Aging of the U.S. Population

	Median Age (Years)
1950	30.2
1970	28.0
1990	34.6
1996	34.6
Projected:	
2000	35.7
2025	38.0
2050	38.1

Source: Reprinted from Statistical Abstract of the United States, p. 14, 1997, Economics and Statistic Administration, U.S. Department of Commerce.

Table 2–2 Ratio of Working-Age Population to the Retirement-Age Population

	1960	1990	2010	2040
United States	6.5	5.3	5.3	3.1
Japan	10.5	5.8	3.4	2.6
United Kingdom	5.6	4.3	4.5	3.0

Source: Data from *International Economic Trends*, © 1996, St. Louis Federal Reserve Bank and Organization for Economic Cooperation and Development.

try. For the United States, the ratio has declined modestly since 1960, and it is projected to decline sharply from 2010 to 2040. The main reason for this is the projected increase in the fraction of the United States population over 65. This share is projected to hold steady at about 12.7% from 1996 to 2000, but it is projected to rise sharply to 20.0% in 2030. (After 2030, the share is projected to level off again through 2050.) Taken by itself, the resulting decline in the support ratio from 2010 to 2030 implies either that the tax burden on the working-age population will have to rise substantially or that benefits to recipients will have to fall substantially, or that some combination of the two must occur.

Physician leaders need to be aware of several factors that will affect favorably the ability of the United States economy to support future retirees. The most important of these is that the productivity of the working-age population is likely to rise strongly over the next 20–40 years. An increase in productivity increases output per worker and real wages per worker and thus can prevent or reduce the necessity of raising the tax *rate* on the future working-age population.

One of the most striking economic phenomena over the past century or more has been the ability of the world's advanced economies to grow over time and, in particular, for output per worker to increase. Table 2–3 shows the performance of three of the world's advanced economies over the long period of 1870–1996 in raising output per capita. Of particular interest is the fact that an apparently modest annual rate of growth, if maintained for sufficiently long periods of time, is capable of raising output per capita by spectacular amounts. For example, the United States growth rate over the period was 1.84%, and this was sufficient to increase output per capita by a factor of 10 over the 126-year period. Further, a difference of only a half percentage point was enough for the United States to surpass and far ex-

Table 2–3 Level and Growth Rates of Per Capita Real GDP, 1870 to 1996

	Level in 1996 U.S. Dollars		Average Annual Growth Rate in Percent		
	1870	*1996*	*1870–1996*	*1955–73*	*1973–96*
United States	2,853	28,554	1.84	2.12	1.50
Japan	937	24,108	2.58	8.07	2.59
United Kingdom	3,665	20,290	1.34	2.48	1.67

Source: Reprinted with permission from R.J. Gordon, *Macroeconomics*, p. 275, © 1997, Addison-Wesley. 1870–1996 GDP data from A. Madison, *Phases of Capitalist Development*, © 1986, Oxford University Press.

ceed the United Kingdom in per capita output. It follows that a critical factor in determining the ability of the United States economy to support the country's Social Security, Medicare, and Medicaid programs in the long run (30 or 40 years) is the rate of output growth that the economy is able to achieve.

As Table 2–3 makes clear, however, maintaining a particular long-run growth rate is not automatic. In the case of the advanced countries, growth since 1973 has been significantly slower than during the earlier post-World War II period. Further, not all countries have positive economic growth rates. The success stories of some of the world's emerging economies (notably South Korea, Taiwan, Malaysia, Thailand, and more recently, Ireland) are well known. However, some low-income countries have suffered declines in output per capita in recent decades, and others have grown so slowly that the gap between their per capita incomes and those of the wealthy nations has increased. Given the importance of growth rates, what factors determine the ability of a country to grow over time? We develop the answer to this question by sketching the essentials of a *model* that economists have long used to analyze long-run growth. Solow (1956) developed the original model. Mankiw, Romer, and Weil refined the original model in 1992 (Mankiw et al., 1992); the refined version is called the "augmented Solow model."

THE SOLOW GROWTH MODEL

A useful tool for analyzing a country's aggregate economy is the concept of the production function. The production function states that a country's output of goods and services depends on the amount of inputs available for use by firms in producing their output. We initially identify two inputs: physical capital (machinery, equipment, and structures) and labor. We designate the amount of output per time period (e.g., per year) as Y, the stock of physical capital as K, and the size of the labor force as L, so that the production function is

$$Y = F(K, L). \tag{1}$$

Equation (1) states that the amount of output that an economy can produce is a function of the amount of resources available. (Income is earned by workers and by the owners of firms in the process of producing output. Therefore, the symbol Y does double duty, representing both output and earned income.)

We initially hold constant the level of technology. We assume that constant returns to scale prevail, so that a doubling of the two inputs results in a doubling of output. This assumption leads to the result that output per worker depends on the amount of capital stock per worker:

$$Y/L = F(K/L). \tag{2}$$

We follow the convention of writing per person variables in lowercase letters, so that Equation (2) becomes

$$y = f(k). \tag{3}$$

That is, a crucial implication of Solow's work is that a country can raise its output per worker by increasing the amount of physical capital per worker. The relation between y and k is shown in Figure 2–2. Note that whereas output per worker is an increasing function of the amount of capital per worker, it is assumed that the increment to output diminishes as k rises.

Saving and Investment

How does a country increase the amount of capital per worker? Given the time path of the country's population growth rate, there is only one way: to increase the fraction of its output that is in the form of physical capital goods. The output of such goods is called investment, and to increase the investment share of output initially requires a reduction in the

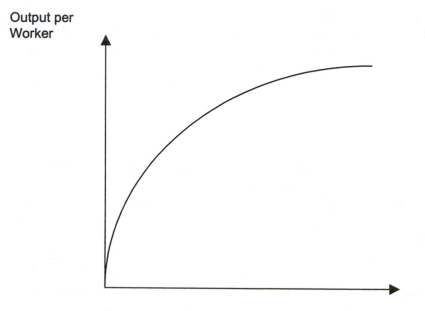

Figure 2–2 Aggregate Production Function with Diminishing Marginal Product of Capital. Marginal product is the increment to output associated with an increase in capital per worker of one unit.

---

share of output devoted to other goods. In particular, a reduction in the share of consumer goods and/or government consumption can achieve a higher investment ratio. A higher current investment ratio implies a larger stock of physical capital per worker in the future.

Increased abstinence from current consumption by households and government implies a higher *national saving rate* in the economy. The national saving rate is defined as

$$s = S/Y, \tag{4}$$

where S is the amount of national saving and Y is aggregate income. National saving comes from three sources: households, business firms, and government. Personal saving is carried out by households; business saving consists of retained earnings and depreciation allowances; and government saving consists of the budget surplus of all levels of government (federal, state, and local) combined.

In the United States, personal saving is low compared to many other countries, amounting to only 3.9% of disposable personal income in 1997. Business saving, however, is much larger than personal saving. Further, government saving has increased dramatically in the United States in recent years. Government saving can be either positive or negative. If annual government revenues exceed annual outlays, government will have a surplus (positive saving). But if revenues fall short of outlays, government will have a deficit (negative saving). A government deficit constitutes negative saving because some portion of private saving must be used to finance the government deficit and therefore is not available to finance private business investment.

National saving in the United States has increased significantly in recent years, rising from about 13% of the gross domestic product (GDP) in 1992 to 18% of GDP in 1997. Much of this increase in the saving rate is attributable to the elimination of the federal budget deficit, which stood at $281 billion in 1992. The federal budget deficit shrank to $29 billion in 1997, and the federal government thus far in 1998 is experiencing a surplus of about $50 billion at an annual rate. State and local governments have achieved surpluses for the last two decades, and the combined surplus for all state and local governments in the United States has been running at a rate of about $70 billion per year in recent years.

In a closed economy (one in which no trade or financial transactions occur with other countries), the financing of new investment requires domestic funds. Consequently, the only way that a country can increase its investment ratio is by raising its domestic saving rate. The augmented Solow model implies that a critical factor affecting the ability of the United States economy to grow strongly in the future (and, by implication, to support its aging population) is the ability to keep the national saving rate near or above the current figure.

In an open economy, a country is not forced to rely solely on domestic saving to finance its domestic investment. Investment in the United States can exceed national saving if wealthholders in the rest of the world are willing and able to purchase financial assets issued by United States firms. This has been a significant source of funds for United States firms during most years of the last two decades. In 1997, gross investment amounted to more than 19% of GDP in the United States, so borrowing from foreigners financed about 1% of United States gross investment. (The opposite situation prevailed in Japan, which had a gross saving rate of 32% in 1996, compared to a gross investment ratio of less than 30%. Japan was financing not only its own investment but also a portion of investment in the rest of the world.)

But foreign borrowing is not really a complete solution for a low domestic saving rate. To the extent that residents of Japan and other countries finance United States investment projects, foreigners (rather than United States residents) receive the future interest and profits from United States investment projects. A superior solution is to achieve and maintain a high domestic saving rate, and the recent performance of the United States economy (especially the elimination of the federal deficit) is a promising step in that direction. Several empirical studies have found a strong positive relation between the national saving rate and per capita income growth. Table 2–4 shows some suggestive evidences for six countries.

Population Growth

Given a country's capital stock, the larger its population, the lower will be its capital-to-labor ratio. Population growth of most advanced countries is low, and thus does not threaten to reduce capital-to-labor ratios in those countries. Excessive population growth, however, is a very real threat in many of the world's poorest countries, and is a major factor in

Table 2–4 Data for Some Individual Countries: The Relation Between National Saving and Economic Growth

Saving Rate > 20%	National Saving as Percent of GDP[a]	Growth in GDP Per Capita[b]
Japan	32.5	5.6
Taiwan	31.4	8.5
Italy	23.4	3.7
Saving Rate < 20%		
Sweden	18.3	2.5
United States	17.7	1.9
United Kingdom	16.8	2.2

[a]Saving rates are for the period 1973–89, except for Taiwan (1980–95).
[b]Growth rates are for the period 1955–90, except for Taiwan (1953–95).
Source: Data from Economic Outlook, © 1991, Organization for Economic Cooperation and Development and E. Liao, Taiwan 2000.

preventing such countries from converging toward the per capita income levels of the advanced nations.

Technical Progress

Advances in technology are a major source of long-run increases in output per worker in the Solow model. Technology is essentially knowledge, and improvements in knowledge permit the introduction of new production processes and new products. A useful way of viewing technical progress is that it raises the *effectiveness* of labor and capital. Consequently, the production functions given in Equations (1) and (3) should be altered to allow for the role of technical progress:

$$Y = \alpha F (K, L), \tag{5}$$

$$y = \alpha f (k), \tag{6}$$

where α represents the level of technology. If technical progress is positive (i.e., knowledge is increasing), α rises over time, and the production function depicted in Figure 2–2 shifts upward, showing that output per worker will be higher at each level of k. A country can increase its output per worker *indefinitely* if α rises over time.

The interaction between technical progress and investment is important in the Solow model. It is frequently the case that, for a firm to take advantage of new technology, it must invest in new equipment. A country that has a high investment ratio will be able to adopt new technology more rapidly than a country with a low investment ratio.

Even though it may be the case that new technology is known to all countries, different countries may nevertheless *choose* different technologies. For example, a poor country with abundant labor and low wage rates may choose a labor-intensive production process, whereas a rich country chooses the latest technology, which may involve a higher capital-to-labor ratio. This may be the case if one compares India and the United States. It is estimated that the effectiveness of labor in India is only about one-twentieth that of the United States

THE AUGMENTED SOLOW MODEL

Empirical studies tend to support the predictions of the Solow model. In particular, statistical studies confirm that countries with high investment ratios and low rates of population growth have higher levels of output per worker than countries with low investment ratios and high population growth rates. However, the model does not perform perfectly. Mankiw et al. found a major difficulty with the model: differences in investment ratios and population growth rates are not able to explain fully the enormous differences in per capita income across countries. Mankiw et al. attributed this shortcoming to the absence of a role for *human capital* (HC) in the basic Solow model.

Inclusion of HC in a growth model may help to explain why some countries are unable to adopt advanced production technologies. In principle, HC should be an increasing function of the level of formal schooling of a country's population, the level of informal and on-the-job training, the stock of health of the work force, and perhaps other characteristics of the population. In practice, it is necessary for the investigator to settle on one or a few proxy variables for HC. In a cross-country study, Mankiw et al. used years of formal schooling as a proxy for the level of HC, and they found that inclusion of this variable greatly improves the ability of the Solow model to explain cross-country differences in output per worker. They dub the resulting model the "augmented Solow model." The aggregate production function becomes

$$Y = \alpha F\,(K, L, HC), \tag{7}$$

and the production function in per worker terms becomes

$$y = \alpha f\,(k, hc), \tag{8}$$

where $hc = HC/L$ = human capital per worker.

There are major implications of the inclusion of the HC variable in a growth model. Recall that the Solow model implies that reduction or elimination of government budget deficits raises the national saving rate and thereby raises output per capita. But some government expenditures increase the amount and quality of formal schooling of the labor force, and other government expenditures (such as those that improve the stock of health of the population) may also improve the nation's stock of HC. Barro (1991) suggested that public spending for education (and defense) should be viewed as an investment rather than as government consumption. In any event, economic growth theory does not imply that governments should reduce public spending indiscriminately. Rather, improving the nation's stock of HC should be a goal that is as important as increasing the saving rate.

In the 1990s, a number of efforts have been made to determine the influence of other macroeconomic variables on a country's growth rate. Garrison and Lee (1995) investigated the role of two such variables: the outward orientation of an economy and the variability of a country's output. In a cross-section study of 67 countries for the period of 1960–1987, they found both influences to be statistically significant. They used as a proxy for the "outward-looking" variable the growth rate of a country's export ratio. (The export ratio is the percent of a country's GDP accounted for by exports.) They find that, holding constant a country's investment ratio, stock of HC and initial level of per capita GDP, an increase in the growth rate of the export ratio raises a country's rate of per capita GDP growth. The reasoning is that an increase in foreign trade forces a country's business firms to be competitive with firms in other countries and thereby raises productivity.

Another important macroeconomic variable, the variability of a country's GDP over time, is measured by the standard deviation of the growth rate of aggregate real GDP (SGY) in the Garrison and Lee (1995) study. Garrison & Lee (1995) found that an increase in SGY lowers a country's long-run growth rate. The reasoning is that higher variability of output (e.g., due to more frequent short-run recessions) raises the uncertainty associated with a firm's future market. This in turn increases the uncertainty associated with the future profitability of current investment projects by the firm. Because overinvestment is costly to the firm, higher SGY reduces current investment. An implication is that if a country can reduce the frequency and severity of recessions, its investment will increase and, in the long run, its ratio of capital to labor will be higher.

Is it possible for a country to select macroeconomic policies that reduce the short-run variability of its aggregate output? If it is possible, a country can improve its long-run growth and achieve a higher ratio of physical capital stock per worker. Because cyclical variability appears to be an important determinant of long-run growth, we next explore the causes of short-run variability and the prospects for alleviating such variability.

REDUCING AGGREGATE VARIABILITY

According to the above analysis, reducing the frequency and severity of recessions is a key to maintaining a high investment ratio and a high long-run rate of economic growth. The United States has a decidedly mixed record in achieving this goal. Since 1953, the United States has experienced eight recessions, several of them quite severe. For example, the unemployment rate rose to at least 7.0% in the recessions of 1957–1958, 1960, 1973–1975, 1980, 1981–1982, and 1991–1992. However, in some decades, the United States economy has avoided recession for as long as 7 years: 1961–1968, 1983–1989, and 1992–1998. Perhaps a cause for optimism is that the United States experienced seven recessions during the period of 1953–1982, but only one recession during the period 1983–1998. What are the prospects that the United States economy will (1) extend the current 7-year period of uninterrupted gains in real output and (2) enjoy favorable cyclical performance well into the next century, with infrequent and mild recessions? Further, what are the conditions necessary for such a desirable performance?

What Causes Recessions?

Business cycle movements are fundamentally different from long-run growth. Whereas long-run growth is measured over several decades or even a century or more, cyclical expansions typically last for only a few years before they are interrupted by a recession. But cyclical expansions do not die of natural causes. Rather, the consensus opinion among economists is that cyclical expansions come to an end only because aggregate demand in the economy declines to a level insufficient to sustain continued increases in output, and consequently a recession occurs. During recessions, the degree of resource utilization declines: the fraction of the labor force employed goes down, and the rate of utilization of the capital stock also falls. During cyclical expansions, aggregate demand rises and the degree of resource utilization goes up. By comparison, long-run growth is characterized by increases in the economy's capacity to produce goods and services. We may think of long-run growth as being driven primarily by forces on the supply side of the economy. On the other hand, most economists view cyclical movements in output as being driven typically by *demand* forces.

It therefore might seem a simple matter to avoid recessions. Why does not the government, including the monetary authority (in the United States, the Federal Reserve), act to increase aggregate demand for goods when a recession threatens? The answer is that government policy makers have not one but two main goals: (1) high output and (2) price stability.

These two goals occasionally may conflict, and the Federal Reserve typically concludes that its main goal is to preserve price stability. A strong case can be made that almost all recessions in the United States since World War II have been due to Federal Reserve actions designed to combat inflation. The conflict arises because inflation typically (but not always) is thought to be due to excessive aggregate demand in the economy. Further, this response of inflation to excessive aggregate demand appears to be a gradual one.

The tool that is available to the Federal Reserve to reduce excessive demand is higher interest rates. The Federal Reserve, through its monetary policies, can raise interest rates and thereby reduce demand for goods. The goal of such monetary restriction is to prevent firms from raising prices as much as they would if demand for their goods were permitted to remain "excessive." The Federal Reserve takes the view that, because the emergence of inflation is a gradual process, failure to take timely action will permit the inflation problem to get worse. Unfortunately, the usual byproduct of restrictive monetary action by the Federal Reserve is an absolute reduction in the economy's output; that is, a recession.

It follows that the key to avoiding recessions is for the economy to avoid situations in which excessive demand will cause, or threaten to cause, inflation. This was obviously difficult to achieve during much of the period from 1953 through 1982. However, the last 15 years present a much more optimistic picture. It is possible that certain developments during the 1980s and 1990s have reduced the extent to which the United States economy, and probably other economies, are susceptible to inflation. To investigate this possibility, we next sketch a model of the way in which firms adjust price in an advanced economy.

INFLATION AND THE PHILLIPS CURVE

Imperfect Competition and Menu Costs

Empirical research strongly supports the conclusion that most firms do not adjust price immediately in the event of a demand shift. Rather, firms appear to change price infrequently (see Blinder, 1991). In the mid-1980s, a number of economists initiated a research agenda, termed the "new Keynesian economics," aimed at answering the following question: In the event of a shift in demand for a firm's output, why does the firm not immediately adjust price? The new Keynesian economists regard this phenomenon as the most important question facing macroeconomics today. As we see below, their analysis leads to the conclusion that the price-output relation is described by a "Phillips curve."

The first ingredient of the new Keynesian approach is to model firms as imperfectly competitive. A long tradition in economics is to use the model of perfect competition in analyzing many economic problems. Whereas it is well known that real-world firms do not fit the requirements of the model of perfect competition, many economists argue that firm behavior is sufficiently close to perfect competition that predictions based on the competitive model are useful. However, the new Keynesian economists contend that the perfectly competitive model leads economists astray when it is used to predict the behavior of prices in the aggregate economy. Consequently, the new Keynesians explicitly build imperfect competition into their models.

The price response of imperfectly competitive firms to a shift in demand for their output turns out to be radically different from the response in a perfectly competitive industry. Due to product differentiation, the imperfectly competitive firm will not lose all of its sales if it fails to reduce price in response to a fall in demand. As a result, the loss to the firm is small if it fails to adjust price. Consequently, a "near-rational" firm will not adjust price but rather will reduce output. On the other hand, a perfectly competitive firm (e.g., a soybean producer) would lose all of its sales if it held out for a price above the market price.

The second ingredient in new Keynesian economics is that there exists a cost to the firm of adjusting price. Critics of the new Keynesian approach point out that such costs are likely to be small. (The cost of changing price is called a "menu cost.") But the gain to the imperfectly competitive firm, if it adjusts price, is also small. If the cost of adjusting price is greater than the gain from adjusting price, even the fully rational firm will not adjust price immediately in the event of a change in demand. Instead, the firm will adjust price infrequently. Among the imperfectly competitive firms studied by Blinder, more than half changed price once per year or less, and three-fourths changed price twice per year or less.

In the new Keynesian model, however, when firms do make price changes, they take into account the direction of any demand changes since their last price change. As a result, price moves in the same direction as output, but price changes in the aggregate economy are gradual rather than instantaneous. Because the unemployment rate moves in the opposite direction as output, there will exist a negative relation between the rate of inflation and the unemployment rate. This negative relation is called the Phillips curve, and it is illustrated in Figure 2–3.

The Phillips curve implies a fairly pessimistic outlook. As unemployment falls during a business cycle expansion, the rate of inflation tends to rise and this in turn risks the possibility that the Federal Reserve will institute a restrictive monetary action. On the other hand, if the Phillips curve can be shifted downward, either through government policies or other events, the need for restrictive monetary action might be avoided. Fortunately, the United States and the other advanced economies of the world appear to have been the beneficiaries of such downward shifts during the 1990s and for a part of the 1980s. These shifts have taken the form of lower inflation for any particular rate of unemployment.

The Shifting Phillips Curve

What have been the forces leading to lower inflation, and can we expect a continuation of these forces in the future? One cause appears to be that

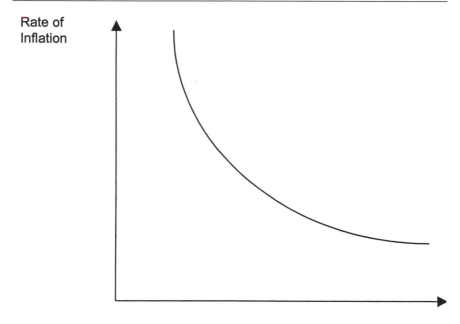

Figure 2–3 The Phillips Curve.

the world is in the midst of an exceptional period of sustained growth in foreign trade among countries, due in part to reduced trade barriers. For instance, United States exports, which were only 4.8% of GDP in 1960, rose to 11.8% of GDP in 1997, and imports rose from 4.3% to 13.1% of GDP during the same period. These trends reduce inflation because firms have less ability to raise prices during cyclical expansions if they must compete not only with domestic rivals but also with foreign firms.

A second cause of lower inflation for a given unemployment rate has been a speedup in the rate of growth of labor productivity during the 1990s. After averaging an annual rate of increase of only about 0.6% from 1978 to 1990, the annual rate of increase of output per worker in the United States rose to 1.2% during the period from 1990 to 1997. More recently, the rate from 1995 to 1997 was 2.0% per year. Productivity increases of this magnitude make it possible for firms to grant wage increases during periods of low unemployment without raising prices.

The reason(s) for the recent impressive gains in productivity are not yet clear. The most likely explanation appears to be the heavy investment in equipment, especially computers, during the 1990s. If this is the case, further investment in computers and in the HC required to use them will permit continuation of productivity improvements.

The decline of union strength, especially in the private sector, may be a source of wage restraint by workers and therefore of price restraint by firms. A negative consequence of the decline in unions may be the increased inequality of incomes in the United States in the last two decades and especially in the 1990s. Inequality, already much higher in the United States than in Europe, has increased sharply since the 1970s. However, the decline in the strength of unions is only one reason for increased inequality. A more fundamental force is probably technological; technical progress has raised the demand for skilled and highly educated workers relative to the demand for unskilled nonsupervisory workers.

Another contributing factor of special interest to physician leaders is the reduction in the rate of increase of health care prices, which is widely attributed to the cost-cutting initiatives of HMOs and related organizations. Until the advent of managed care, there was little or no incentive for patients, hospitals, and physicians to hold down medical expenditures. The health care sector accounts for about 14% of GDP, and it is large enough to have a perceptible effect on the aggregate price level. Finally, the advanced economies of the world have been the beneficiaries of falling prices of oil during the mid-1980s and again in 1997–1998. Oil is so important as a fuel that a decline in its price is sufficient to exert downward pressure on the aggregate rate of inflation.

The forces discussed above have combined to shift the Phillips curve downward in the 1990s (see Figure 2–4). As a consequence, the Federal Reserve has not deemed it necessary to restrict demand, and the economy has been recession-free. The absence of recessions has reduced the variability of output and encouraged investment in new capital goods. A continuation of these forces will keep the Phillips curve "low" or perhaps shift it downward even further. If this can be accomplished, economic growth will reduce significantly the need for future tax increases to support our Social Security, Medicare, and Medicaid programs.

A useful measure of the ability of society to support these programs in the future is per capita real GDP (PCGDP). As noted in Table 2–3, the United States achieved an average annual growth rate of 1.5% for PCGDP during the period of 1973–1996. If this rate of growth can be maintained, PCGDP will increase from $28,554 in 1996 to $47,400 in 2030 and to $55,000 in 2040 (figures are in 1996 $). That is, per capita output of the U.S. economy (in real terms) would be 93% higher in 2040 than in 1996. Growth of this magnitude would contribute substantially to the ability of the United States working population to support the retired population in the future and thereby would help to offset the decline in the ratio of working-age population to retirement-age population between now and 2040 (see Table 2–2).

However, it should be noted that there is no guarantee that the forces that have led to long-run economic growth in the past will lead to similar rates of growth in the future. Achieving a strong rate of future growth will depend on two crucial requirements:

1. It is important for the United States to maintain a low frequency and severity of recessions. This will provide an environment conducive to strong investment in physical capital by business firms. In turn, the ability to avoid recessions will depend on keeping inflation low. Recessions can be avoided only if the Federal Reserve does not have to intervene in the economy to fight excessive inflation. This scenario can be achieved if the forces that have tended to reduce inflation recently will continue to be as strong in the next century. Reversal of these forces could cause the prospects for avoiding serious recessions in the next century to vanish.

2. It is essential for the United States to maintain a strong national saving rate to promote investment and continued growth of income

Rate of
Inflation

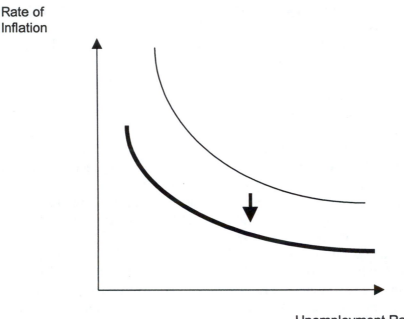

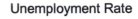

Unemployment Rate

Figure 2–4 A Downward Shift of the Phillips Curve. When the curve shifts downward, inflation is lower at any particular rate of unemployment.

and output per capita. In particular, it is highly desirable for the federal government to avoid returning to the era of budget deficits. Large budget deficits absorb private saving that otherwise could be used to finance investment in new physical capital by business firms. A source of concern is that the ratio of working-age population to retired population will decline sharply after 2010. To prepare for this demographic event, the recent improvement in the national saving rate must be maintained.

GLOSSARY

business cycle. a decline in aggregate output of goods and services, followed by an expansion in aggregate output.

closed economy. a country that does not engage in trade of goods, services, or financial assets with other countries.

depreciation. the reduction in the value of a country's stock of physical capital goods due to wearing out and obsolescence.

economic growth. sustained growth in the productive capacity of an economy.

exports. goods and services produced in the domestic economy and sold to residents of other countries.

government budget deficit. the excess of government expenditures over tax revenues, usually stated at an annual rate.

government budget surplus. the excess of government tax revenues over expenditures, usually stated at an annual rate.

gross domestic product (GDP). the value of all goods and services produced in a country during a particular time period.

human capital. a type of capital embodied in a country's work force. A nation's accumulation of human capital occurs as a result of investment in education, health, and training.

imperfect competition. a market in which sellers have some degree of monopoly power; that is, firms are "price setters." A possible source of such monopoly power is that the output of one seller is "differentiated" from the output of other sellers; that is, goods are heterogeneous.

imports. goods purchased by individuals and firms in the domestic economy but produced in other countries.

inflation. a rise in a country's average price level. The inflation rate is the percentage rate of change in the average price level, expressed at an annual rate.

investment. the part of GDP that either adds to a country's stock of physical capital goods or replaces worn-out physical capital goods.

menu cost. a cost to the firm of adjusting the price at which it sells a good or service.

national saving. the sum of personal saving by households, business saving by corporations, and public saving by government.

new Keynesian economics. a school of thought that attempts to explain inflexibility of goods prices and wage rates as an outcome of firms' profit-maximizing behavior.

open economy. a country that sells exports to other nations, buys imports from firms located in other countries, and engages in exchange of assets with residents of other countries.

perfect competition. a market in which agents are so small that no single buyer or seller can exert a perceptible influence on price. Further, the good or service produced must be homogeneous. As a result, sellers are "price takers."

personal saving. the portion of personal income that is not spent for consumption nor paid out to government as taxes.

Phillips curve. the negative relation between the rate of inflation and the rate of unemployment.

physical capital. structures and equipment used in the production process.

production function. the relation between output and the inputs used in the production process.

productivity. the amount of output produced per worker or per hour.

real GDP. the value of a country's output (gross domestic product) in constant prices.

recession. a decline in aggregate output in an economy; that is, the phase of the business cycle between a peak and a trough.

REFERENCES

Barro, R. (1991). Economic growth in a cross section of countries. *Quarterly Journal of Economics, 106,* 407–443.

Blinder, A. (1991). Why are prices sticky? Preliminary results from an interview study. *American Economic Review, 81,* 89–96.

Garrison, C., & Lee, F.-Y. (1995). The effect of macroeconomic variables on economic growth rates: A cross-country study. *Journal of Macroeconomics, 17,* 303–317.

Mankiw, N.G., Romer, D., & Weil, D.N. (1992). A contribution to the empirics of economic growth. *Quarterly Journal of Economics, 107,* 407–437.

Solow, R. (1956). A contribution to the theory of economic growth. *Quarterly Journal of Economics, 70,* 65–94.

CHAPTER 3

Health Policy for the Physician Leader

Curtis P. McLaughlin

TABLE OF CONTENTS

EXECUTIVE SUMMARY

This chapter discusses the reasons why physician leaders in an executive MBA program would become involved in a course in health policy. It describes one such course and how it integrates with other courses in such a curriculum. This is presented through consideration of a number of key health policy questions, including the following:

- Just exactly where are we?
- How did we get here?
- Do we want to be there?
- What other alternatives are there throughout the world?
- What is likely to work in the future?
- How do we prepare for it, given our political process?
- What is the likely role of physician leaders in this process?
- How can such roles be enhanced?

These questions motivate physician managers and leaders starting with a historical perspective and addressing a number of future policy questions.

This chapter then outlines six types of risks to be managed at an organizational and societal level: (1) underwriting, (2) marketing, (3) clinical operations, (4) financial, (5) regulatory, and (6) integrative. These are then used to review the following questions:

- Which of these risks am I comfortable handling?
- Which other ones do I need and want to learn to handle?
- How can I use this program to learn to handle those risks that I need and want to learn to handle?

While potential physician leaders may be used to answering these questions for their individual practices, they seldom have had experience dealing with them in the context of large health care organizations, communities, or whole societies. This discussion motivates many of the understandings and skills covered in the health policy course, including (1) defining managerial risks in complex situations, (2) selecting and evaluating technological alternatives, (3) understanding the Alphabet Soup of organizational forms being offered to structure future health care, (4) the current roles of physician leaders in managing these structures, and (5) assessing and self-selecting one's future personal role in developing health policy for a large organization, community, or society.

This chapter then concludes with a discussion of how these skills can be augmented through the process of an executive MBA involving distance learning — through preparation, skills development, networking, and practicing leadership during one's concurrent employment.

An MBA program does not usually include a required course in health policy, although related issues of microeconomics, regulation, the influence of society on business, and business ethics are commonly addressed by MBA programs. For physician leaders these issues are especially relevant today because of (1) the high uncertainty associated with the rapidly changing health care environment and (2) the high likelihood of further government regulation affecting health care organizations. Therefore, a physician-oriented MBA needs to address those issues in the context of health care.

Integration

The health policy course can be conceived of as part of the managerial role of dealing with the external environment. It integrates with concepts studied in the strategy and marketing courses. These deal respectively with (1) describing the external environment in a dynamic political and social sense (health policy); (2) deciding on how the organization will respond competitively to this environment (strategy); and (3) how the organization will measure and influence the needs and desires of this environment (marketing). Obviously, all of these have a strong microeconomic component as well, so these three courses need to interact strongly with the economics course and with the influence of those economics on the availability of capital resources (finance) and of people resources (organizational behavior). In a program carefully tailored for physicians there can also be strong links to the topics of disease management, quality management, and information technology.

KEY QUESTIONS OF HEALTH POLICY

One might worry that having physicians study health policy is like carrying coal to Newcastle. Any such course would have to enter territory that the participants inhabit day and night. However, the objective of such a course in an Executive MBA for physicians is not familiarization, but precision in thinking about something that one might believe to be familiar. It addresses questions such as the following:

- Just exactly where are we?
- How did we get here?
- Do we want to be there?
- What other alternatives are there throughout the world?
- What is likely to work in the future?
- How do we prepare for it, given our political process?
- What is the likely role of physician leaders in this process?
- How can such roles be enhanced?

Can we expect the assembled participants to agree on the answers to those questions? Of course not. Our goal is to help the participants develop an objective, managerial approach to decision-making with precise definitions of terms and relationships and careful consideration of both sides of key issues and points-of-view before reaching individual conclusions. One objective of most adult management education is to give the participants an array of alternative tools for interpreting and analyzing events, situations and alternatives, tools to use in addition to the approaches that they have already developed through their professional and managerial experience. They should not be asked to abandon what has worked, but to develop a toolkit that allows them to perform as well or better using a broader array of approaches to fit a wider variety of situations.

Where Are We?

The health care environment is undergoing massive restructuring. Managed care has become the dominant form of organization of care delivery. Practices and institutions are merging or selling out to a wide array of health care organizations. Physician incomes, especially those of specialists, are dropping rapidly. These are all symptoms of the industrialization of what has been a cottage industry organized along craft lines, despite being 13 to 14% of our country's economic activity. Therefore, the course must include a framework for interpreting and finding a desired endpoint for this industrialization process. We have chosen to use the Boynton, Victor and Pine (1993) model of stages of industrialization—craft to mass production to continuous improvement to mass customization. We emphasize that mass production does exist in areas such as cataract surgery and other "Centers of Excellence," but that there is a widespread desire to avoid mass production of services that is legitimate given the high inherent variability in patient anatomy, physiology and psychological needs and preferences. Mass customization is emphasized as the logical end point for this process. Health care is a mixture of art and science and our course looks at the consequences of matches and mismatches between situations high in art that fit with craft (apprenticeship and job costing or fee-for-service) and those high in science which fits with industrialization (bundled payments, use of clinical pathways, length-of-stay controls). This industrialization model can be supported by readings published by this author (1998) and by the Kongstvedt text (1997).

These rapid changes conflict with stable professional values concerning personal and professional autonomy, authority and leadership. Therefore, the health policy course has to focus early on professional versus organizational conflicts and allow physician participants to understand the interaction between the two—the profession and the organization. Today these interactions often focus around ownership of intellectual capital. Health care has historically assumed that this resided with the professional. Because of issues of economies of scale, much of the cost of developing this knowledge was borne by the federal government through National Institutes of Health (NIH), Agency for Health Care Policy and Research (AHCPR), and Centers for Disease Control and Prevention (CDC). However, industrialization and its accompanying mergers and networks has resulted in units of sufficient institutional size and scope to support proprietary R&D in areas beyond pharmaceuticals and medical devices. Competition increasingly depends on the development of best practices by an institution and their rapid dissemination and adoption by the bulk of the practitioners in the system. Organizational learning becomes the focus of organizational processes. That raises new questions about federal and state government policies, about support for research, for continuing medical graduate medical education, and access to clinical records and research outputs. Participants must be prepared to take leadership positions in debating these issues.

How Did We Get Here?

There is a saying that those who fail to learn from history are doomed to repeat it. Therefore, an MBA program should address the history of health care financing and policymaking in the United States. This could start with the Tenth Amendment to the United States Constitution, which states that those powers not expressly given to the federal government belong to state and local governments. Health and education were not expressly given to the federal government in the Constitution. However, federal involvement can be argued for under the welfare clause of Constitution and also through Jefferson's argument of implied powers. The way that this has played out is that with minor exceptions the federal government has financed national programs of health and education, but not tried to deliver the services directly. At times the federal government has taken a planning role or used the carrot-and-stick approach. The latter can be exemplified by withholding highway funds, if conditions on speed limits and vehicle inspections are not met by an individual state. However, this constitutional reality has constrained us whenever we have attempted to consider seriously a national health policy. While the debate over the Clinton Health Plan became a battle of interest groups, we also have to recognize that the debate took place within a context that called into question the power of the federal government to take a more activist role.

One could go back centuries to medical care as a religious calling and not a scientific field—to when the term hospice was much more representative than hospital. However, in a business school it makes sense to start by focusing on how the delivery and financing of health care in the United States became so closely linked to one's employment status, rather than to citizenship or to membership in humanity. Therefore, we suggest starting with the system of combined fee-for-service and charity care that existed prior to World War II and tracing the development and gradual introduction of such elements as group health insurance and prepaid group practices into a system in which physicians initially took what people could pay and teaching institutions provided free care in return for allowing learners to work on those who could not pay. The Blue Cross/Blue Shield systems were started in the Great Depression to try to stabilize the cash flows to the providers.[1] World War II saw the industrialization of all available hands, breaking the Great Depression, and giving rise to the power of industrial unions and to the era of big science. It also led to optimism that collectively Americans could accomplish anything that they wanted to (Strauss & Howe, 1991).

During World War II, wage and price controls were imposed. Later on, as the workers became restless for better compensation, the Office of

---

[1] Prepaid group practices, known today as Health Maintenance Organizations (HMOs), were also started about the same time in response to the same needs for stable cash flows, but remained a relatively minor factor for a number of decades.

Price Administration decided to hold the line on wages, but to allow the granting of improved fringe benefits through collective bargaining. This led to the rapid expansion of health insurance among unionized industrial and government workers. This was also consistent with the provision of medical benefits to the vast military establishment.

Because collective bargaining was the vehicle for determining health benefits and union officials were elected by their membership, union leaders did not choose catastrophic coverage, but sought to maximize the visibility of benefits to their rank-and-file members. This led them to bargain for first-dollar, fee-for-service coverage for everyone and to put limitations on the lifetime benefits for those who were born with or developed catastrophic or high-cost chronic conditions. It also led them to emphasize dependent coverage. They wanted most union members to see something paid frequently out of that benefit.

When Medicare and Medicaid were developed as part of the Great Society, these two programs started out mirroring the structure of health insurance in the industrial sector, but without the lifetime limitations. Neither of these programs dealt with adequate coverage for long-term care nor encouraged prevention and Medicare still does not cover prescription drugs. Because many individuals covered under Medicare and Medicaid had been receiving some form of charity care, the net effect of these programs was to pay for services that had been provided free or at discounts. This increased physician incomes without increasing the supply and increased the demand for services not provided previously. In addition, heavy investments in medical research increased the variety, cost and effectiveness of what providers could do for patients. Thus there was a rapid inflation in prices due to a limited supply and a rapid increase in volume due to technology followed by increases in the supply of providers and facilities available, with these capacity expansions often subsidized by the federal government.

First, the Blues and then the federal government began to exert pressures on their providers, receiving substantial discounts in return for their business. This led to the phenomenon of cost shifting in which private insurers were asked to pay more to cover uncompensated care and other items not covered by the Blues and federal programs. Employers fought back as their premiums jumped at rates well above overall inflation and as foreign competition that did not provide such benefits ate into their markets. They demanded that insurance companies begin to control premiums through various techniques attributed to managed care. These points are supported by a number of readings on the history of United States health care (Kongstvedt, 1997; Mayer & Mayer, 1985; Starr, 1982)

Do We Want To Be There?

In a country that does not have a health policy, it is useful to allow some debate about this question. For physician leaders it is partly a matter of personal taste and partly motivation for studying the merits of the various delivery and payment alternatives available today in the United States and elsewhere. If the instructor has considerable international experience and finds that participants tend to focus a little too closely on the domestic or local situation (e.g., on TennCare), it is possible to shift that focus by looking at the international health scene in collaboration with both the Economics and Strategy courses. This can help raise the discourse to a more macro level.

For example, one can study the case of a prestigious Finnish orthopedic hospital, the Orton Hospital (Masalin, 1994), which outlines the plight of an institution in a different but still rapidly changing environment. In an attempt to reduce government deficits, the Finnish federal government decentralized the administration of its jointly financed government health care program to local governments. These local governments then attempted to control the rising cost of health care by reducing referrals to central specialized hospitals. The Orton Hospital then downsized and reached out to private pay individuals in the Helsinki area. This case can also be used in a Strategy course. This can be buttressed by a reading from a Health Economics book (such as Phelps, 1997 on "General Considerations for a National Health Policy") in which specific questions are raised and comparative data provided from a number of countries including the United States and Finland. This allows participants to consider the components of a national health policy, explicit or implicit, and how countries have handled these components and the impact of these policies on their delivery of care. This reading offers comparisons of per capita health and income, life expectancy, perinatal mortality in many countries, and comparisons of health system characteristics in the United States, Canada, Germany, and Japan. It also outlines the linkages between these variables or lack thereof in these populations. With such data available, educated physicians can join the debate about where the United States wants to go, which can be continued in this course, in the Strategy course, and in Marketing and Economics classes.

What Alternatives Are Out There?

The alternatives are many. There is the whole Alphabet Soup of United States health care out there—HMOs, IPAs, PPOs, POSs, MOSs, etc. However, physician leaders must look carefully at their definitions and characteristics and at their pros and cons, both in terms of currently accepted wisdom and analytically. A text with a glossary, such as Kongstvedt (1997), can help a lot. However, evaluation of the alternatives calls for a bit more detail than this book allows. This calls for an understanding of the types of risks that health care organizations and health care managers may choose to handle or not handle in the design of their system. These have been discussed by this author elsewhere (McLaughlin, 1997; McLaughlin & Kaluzny, 1997). There these risks are defined as underwriting, marketing, clinical operations, financial, regulatory, and integrative risk sets. One focus of this effort is to start participants thinking through the following questions:

- Which of these risks am I now comfortable handling?
- Which other ones do I need and want to learn to handle?
- How can I use this program to learn to handle those that I want or need to handle?

While individual physicians may be used to answering these questions in the context of their individual practices, they seldom have experience dealing with them in the context of large organizations, communities, or societies.

This discussion can serve as motivation for deciding what individual physician leaders need to know and learn about business skills and activities. Then one can analyze the various organizational forms used for health care delivery in terms of how they allocate these important types of risks and how they facilitate their handling. This can be supported by the study of the life cycles of health care organizations and health care markets. This subject can also be addressed in the Strategy course and common case material can be used in both courses. Market cycles can be defined using the cyclical models of either Shortell et al. (1996) or Coile (1997). Participants can also study the life cycle of clinical practices outlined by McLaughlin, Pathman, and Konrad (1997). These risks can also map relatively well on the study of the balanced scorecard in the Accounting course.

The study of Organizational Behavior can also focus on the role of the governance process in the operation of these various alternative organizational forms. Health care professionals guard and maintain the technological core health care organizations. They demand a role in its governance processes and governance mechanisms that are keys to effective technical and organizational change. This also provides motivation for later study of roles for medical directors in the governance of health care organizations and in development of health policy for the organization, its patients, and the communities in which it operates.

Many undifferentiated MBA programs are likely to emphasize the importance of publicly-held companies, since considerable wealth can be created by developing a company and taking it public. However, once the company goes public, it is beholden primarily to one set of stakeholders, its stockholders. Therefore, there is still a major role in health care for the not-for-profit organization that does not respond only to stockholders, but can balance a large number of competing interests. Therefore, a deeper knowledge of not-for-profit organizations and their behaviors are necessary for determining their role in setting and implementing health policy. This is especially true of the entrepreneurial not-for-profit organization, which can be as full a participant in the marketplace as a stock corporation, provided it does not need to raise large amounts of equity capital quickly. The participant must understand the similarities and differences in how these two types of organizations function. The term often applied to the roles of management, staff, and boards in both for-profit and not-for-profit organizations is governance. Physician leaders must be able to function and help govern effectively in one or the other or both.

How they handle risks:

Between these conceptualizations of risks to be encountered, organizational forms available for delivery of care, and life cycles of local markets and delivery organizations, plus the other concepts acquired in Strategy and Marketing courses, physician leaders become equipped to analyze their local health care systems, preferably including the organizations they work in. They also can have the opportunity to practice these skills and concepts on cases such as the Orton Hospital and Mt. Auburn Hospital cases. They can practice in the context of a written assignment to analyze an altogether different community and a different set of health care services, such as in the County Physical Therapy, Caribou, ME (Ezzy & Scott, 1995) case. This is about the delivery of physical therapy (PT) services in a sparsely settled remote rural area and how a successful practitioner of PT should organize his or her practice in the future. Participants can be asked to analyze the community in terms of the stages described by Coile (1997) or by Shortell et al. (1996) to identify the drivers in the situation, compare it to their own experience base, and to make sense in writing of the situation in the case. The instructor can offer feedback on the analysis and the student can then be charged with writing a planning recommendation for the PT practitioner in the case based on the analysis. Participants can also be encouraged to use the risk categories discussed earlier in analyzing and justifying their recommendations. This two-stage, interactive format is suggested when participating physicians do not have experience writing case analyses. Early feedback can keep them on track and motivated in the analysis and recommendations. Good expository writing skills are necessary, because large organizations depend to a large degree on the circulation of written plans, proposals, and analyses for decision making.

Planning Alternatives:

Physician leaders must be able to analyze issues of health care policy for specific communities and specific segments of health care. These have to be analyzed against specific public health criteria of quality, access, and cost. Here the health policy course intersects with the courses that cover issues of quality and quality improvement. However, one can also begin to focus on one of the risks to be managed, underwriting (including pricing). Participants can read about issues such as managed behavioral health care services and about rating and underwriting. They also should have supporting sessions on quality measurement and improvement and on disease management. For example, we sometimes use a case on contracting for behavioral health care services in Seattle, Washington (Ilinitch & McLaughlin, 1998), which raises all types of issues of public health and health policy as it relates to managed care for disadvantaged populations. It also brings home issues of the impact of mismatches between the low science segments of health care and the specificity required for effective managed care. It raises a number of issues about the privatization of public health care in the United States. Here the author of this chapter has been able to provide some insights on the privatization issue based on Halverson, Kaluzny, and McLaughlin's *Public Health and Managed Care* (1998). The Nash County Hospital case from that book also allows one to consider objectively the various viewpoints on the privatization of public health care facilities (McLaughlin, 1998b).

Imbedded in such studies are opportunities to develop insights about the ability or inability of organizations to handle high levels of inherent variability in definitions, patients, events, costs, etc. This needs to be a continuing theme in the health policy course, one relating back to the issues of art versus science and Deming's notions about special cause variation and common cause variation (1986). The administration of health care has historically treated an art form as if it were a science and assumed that any negative consequences were the result of special cause variation, that is, held the individual practitioner responsible for adverse events. What future managers have to learn from the Deming approach is that this will be a field that even without special cause variation will have high variability and that administrative systems have to be tailored to that reality. As Deming would say, "The system is the problem," to which we would add, "especially if it fails to handle inherent variability fairly and effectively." Physician leaders must come to understand that assessing and adapting to this inherent variability is a key element of the physician-manager's role in health care delivery whether it is organized for craft or mass customization.

Another set of skills that physician leaders must develop pertains to the community as a unit of analysis for health policy. If we are to manage populations rather than just individuals, we must have a sense of how that can be done in and by a community. This author uses a set of readings on the historical development of a community-based health care quality initiative in Kingsport, TN. This is a three – document sequence starting with a case followed by two successive descriptive articles from the *Joint Commission Journal of Quality Management* (McLaughlin & Simpson, 1994; McLaughlin, 1995; McLaughlin, 1998b). This allows us to follow events in this community for some twelve years. These cases show the roles of the human resources managers of the dominant employer, of the two-hospital, of the shared-medical-staff structure of services, of the impact on trust and relationships of various efforts at organizing managed care, and of the limits of community cooperation and planning in a market-driven health care system. It also raises issues of what is proprietary information for competition and what is needed data for public health improvement.

What Is Likely To Work in the Future?

One very important role for the physician leader is as a member of a team that does policy analysis for health care. Such teams require a wide range of skills including management, economics, operations, and medicine. As the owners of the technological core of medicine, physicians can always claim a place at the table. However, they must also be prepared to contribute to the overall progress of process analysis and improvement efforts. Their participation is enhanced by a number of skills typically studied in an MBA program, including how to lead teams, how to analyze processes, how to implement change, and how to evaluate outcomes.

One potential contribution of a health policy course is in the arena of technology assessment. The basic tools of technology assessment involve benefit and cost analysis. However, these are frequently bypassed by health care professionals because of measurement difficulties. These measurement issues pertain primarily to benefits, but also to costs. Analysts crossing over from other industries will find very specific problems in applying their methods of analysis in health care. These problems pertain to lack of cooperation due to fear of loss of autonomy, accounting systems biased toward revenue rather than cost-finding, high levels of inherent variability, compartmentalization of information systems, and poorly aligned reward systems and outcome responsibilities. Effective benefit/cost analysis in health care requires understanding of nomenclature and coding systems used in this industry, effective prediction of risks, experience at analyzing high variability systems, and appropriate stratification of the populations being studied. Furthermore, rampant market failure in this industry has led to the necessity of measuring separately the consumer satisfaction and benefit/cost impacts of specific technological alternatives.

The role of benefit and cost analysis in health care was investigated thoroughly in the 1960s and 70s (Baker et al., 1970; Weinstein & Stason, 1977; Bunker et al., 1979; Office of Technology Assessment, 1980). During that period, the problems of benefit measurement seemed so insurmountable that most health care professionals doing analysis preferred to rely on cost-effectiveness analysis defined by Weinstein and Stason (1977) as

> The key distinction is that a benefit-cost analysis must value all outcomes in economic (e.g., dollar) terms, including lives or years of life and morbidity, whereas a cost-effectiveness analysis serves to place priorities on alternative expenditures without requiring that the dollar value of life and health be presented.

The underlying premise of cost-effectiveness analysis in health problems is that, for any given level resources available, society (or the jurisdiction involved) wishes to maximize the total aggregate health benefits conferred. Alternatively, for a given health-benefit goal, the objective is to minimize the cost of achieving it. In either formulation, the analytical methodology is the same. (p. 717)

Mathematically, one can either maximize the benefits subject to a constraint on costs or minimize costs for a given set of benefits, but not both. However, one finds that the basic problem is not one of using dollars, but one of expressing all relevant factors in any single metric. The alternative approach is to express outcomes as a vector, but since one alternative vector seldom dominates the other, one must still deal with tradeoffs among variables.

The management of technology in health care has a number of requirements that make it different from most industrial decision making. It does not just deal with dollars and cents but with a number of aspects of well-being and occasionally with matters of life and death. Furthermore, health care is an industry undergoing a rapid transition, one in which the basic units for analysis have been shifting from the cost of a visit or a day in the hospital toward the cost of an episode of care or cost per person per period of time, either generally or in population segments or in high-risk groups. McLaughlin and Simpson (1998) have discussed the new realities in technology assessment as analysis has shifted from being demand-driven to become concerned with cost minimization, consumer satisfaction, and adequacy of care and outcomes.

Segmentation:

Health care practices and institutions provide a wide variety of products. Current practice using Diagnosis-related groups (DRG) categories identifies almost 500 products and that differentiation is often too coarse for technological planning. This leads to two requirements for technology management: (1) methods to identify the affected population segments, and (2) simplicity in approach to allow application to many product lines. Not only does one need to have large clinical data bases to identify enough cases affected by a specific technology, but one must also deal with ever-shifting definitions of disease states as medical knowledge accumulates and as the technology, itself, affects the nature and distribution of what is to be treated. An example is the treatment of AIDS. The usual classification schemes differentiate between patients with T-cell counts of 200 or more and those with 100 or less. Portela (1995) found the economic impact of AIDS to be greatest in the population with T-cell counts below 50 and recommended a different segmentation for treatment planning and costing. Since then, however, success with drug "cocktails" involving expensive prophylactic treatment for the much larger population with T-cell counts less than 400 has changed the nature of the disease from one of avoiding overwhelming infections to one of fighting drug toxicity involving much different technical requirements, morbidity patterns, and survival rates.

Technology Assessment Skill Requirements

The MBA health policy course, therefore, should review the combination of clinical assessment skills, data analysis skills and technology evaluation skills needed to assess and implement medical technology, including:

1. Identifying populations affected by the technology: This population must be very carefully defined so that data on it can be mined from available data bases. They must be the population specifically affected by the technology under consideration.
2. Identifying the impact of the technology on treatment of those populations: This usually requires a detailed process analysis, including the identification of the process changes effected by the new technology.
3. Developing detailed protocols for application of that technology: Only by delving into the details can physician managers help estimate the impact of an innovation on costs. These costs are not only monetary but also convenience costs of use for both providers and patients.
4. Projecting outcomes using this proposed best practice: There has to be a visible improvement in health outcome with a new technology. In many countries, clinical improvement must be significant to justify adoption.
5. Projecting degree of adoption and/or compliance with best practice: Physician managers can help identify the drivers that will lead to adoption of a specific protocol by the relevant provider community, taking into account motivation for adoption in both provider and patient communities.

6. Projecting clinical outcomes under a representative cross-section of payment and reward systems: Because we have a mixed payment system, we are likely to see mixed effects from adopting a new technology unless it clearly dominates existing technology on the cost, convenience, and/or health outcomes dimensions.
7. Projecting costs to specific actors under a representative cross-section of payment and reward systems: At present, improved costs are a hurdle that any technology must pass, unless there is a significant and obvious improvement in outcomes and/or quality of life.
8. Comparing results with existing methods of delivery and competing new alternatives: If the multidimensional results are mixed, as they so often are, then determine the tradeoffs between cost, convenience, and outcome quality.
9. Recommending whether to adopt a proposed technology, how best to implement it, and how best to arrange for its adoption and diffusion: Making a recommendation is only the start of the process of technological change. Health care organizations are notoriously slow to change. Given the risks to patients of any change, this is not just resistance to change. There has to be either a significant improvement in cost or outcome and/or a strong understanding of the scientific causation behind the change to see it adopted on any wide scale.

An alternative conceptual approach is provided in Siran and Leffel's chapter on "Quality Management in Managed Care" in Kongstvedt (1997).

It should be clear to the reader that many of the skills involved in technological assessment and professional leadership can also be addressed in courses elsewhere in an integrated MBA curriculum. They are especially relevant to offerings in Operations Management, Disease Management, Quality Improvement, and Information Technology.

How Do We Prepare for It, Given Our Political Process?

Physician participation in the political process is earned through leadership in the medical profession, in medical institutions, and by providing leadership in one's community. Therefore, participants should be asked to look at the roles that physicians now fulfill, especially in managed care. Very little has been written so far about these roles and a great deal of mythology, much of it unrealistic, circulates in the profession. We at Tennessee have already embarked on a case-writing effort to address this weakness in the available teaching materials. In the meantime, we have installed some experiential efforts to make up for this lack of theory and research.

We have already discussed studying the community-based side of decision-making and influence by focusing on the situation in Kingsport, TN. However, there the role of medical leadership was overshadowed by that of corporate leaders, especially corporate benefits managers. However, we did witness the emergence of new physician leaders in specific efforts related to smoking cessation, driver training, care for the uninsured, and fitness training, all at the grass-roots level. What is needed is further understanding of the role of physician leadership in the corporate setting, where the corporation is a provider or insurer. One can deal with this lack of teaching materials by asking the participants to interview individuals who are fulfilling such a role and comparing and contrasting the results. From this process, physician leaders can prepare themselves for a variety of leadership experiences built on a base of facts, skills, and sufficient confidence to achieve results.

What Is the Likely Role of Physician Leaders in This Process?

In response to this question, one can return to a number of earlier learnings and to additional case studies, such as a study of the role of Dr. David Levy in Corning-Franklin Health Group (B) (McLaughlin and Tillman, 1995) and issues addressed in the Harvard case, South Eye Institute (Adams & Herzlinger, 1993). There are many successful physician leaders and some unsuccessful ones. Recent events have shown us situations where successful physician leadership has been followed by failure (Columbia/HCA, FPA) as leaders strayed from their areas of expertise and listened not to their customers, but to those who were concerned only with their stocks' values.

A health policy course can also prepare one for this debate by reviewing the alternative scenarios provided by scholars. One can debate the consumer-oriented free-market approach of Herzlinger (1997) versus the community-based planning approach of Shortell et al. (1996) versus the regulatory approaches being undertaken by the various states. These offer a number of justifiable intellectual positions and leadership roles for suitably trained physicians.

How Can Such Roles Be Enhanced?

We believe that such roles can be enhanced by a number of topics considered in an Executive MBA program that includes a health policy course. These enhancements can take place in a number of ways, including the following:

By Preparation:

The Executive MBA offers the physician the opportunity to adapt to roles above and beyond those associated with clinical care. In case after case, the potential leader had to walk in the shoes of those who are leading, to consider the multiple sides of the issues, to use hard facts and fit them into conceptual and mathematical models that allow one to reduce and refine the array of available alternatives, and select and implement those that are likely to succeed in that environment. At the same time, the health policy course should invite potential leaders to step back from the narrow professional, to see the changes in health care more in the sweep of time and develop a sense of which risks each individual is willing to manage by disposition, position, and circumstance. It can enable the physician leader to think in terms not just of one's professional persona, but also in terms of what is best for society. It also serves as a bulwark against being swept along with fads.

By Skills Development:

This is what an executive MBA is all about. The leader must understand the financial implications of what is being discussed, think in terms of markets and competition, adjust to social, economic, and political change as they play out in United States society, analyze and optimize processes, motivate individuals and teams, etc. All of these move in the direction of exhibiting competence, demonstrating mastery, and gaining respect of one's peers and colleagues, so that one can become eligible to be a contributor on a top management team.

By Networking:

One intriguing part of the executive MBA experience is that the program itself takes place in a virtual network of participants, instructors, facilities, and studies. One learns in the process of surviving how to function in this new professional world. One sees how influence is exerted, nationally, locally, and in one's work group, by knowing when to speak up and when to hold back, when to be the advocate and when to be the analyst, and how to support and move forward the multidisciplinary team, the key element of health care leadership for many years to come. The Internet provides many new opportunities for learning, for gathering data, for influencing others, and for collective effort that holds great promise. Any program based on it can give much hands-on experience with this emerging technology of management and care-giving.

By Practicing Leadership:

If the program is oriented toward physician leadership, the participating physician should have many opportunities to experiment with leadership roles with program peers inside and outside the formal learning setting. When the physician is able to work at a job in parallel with the program, he or she will be able to try out learnings and concepts as they become familiar and then compare experiences with colleagues in the program. Modern communication can provide ample opportunity to share work experiences with the faculty and think about how to proceed in such situations in the future. What participants will find over the course of the year is that leadership tasks at work will come to you as much as you seek them out. Buttressed by the knowledge and skills gained in the course, he or she should be able gradually to assume leadership based on competency and commitment to personal and institutional change. It will not be a case of waiting to graduate to put that new knowledge to use.

GLOSSARY

collective bargaining. the process of negotiation between employers and labor unions resulting in a contractual relationship covering wages and benefits.

continuous improvement. a structured organizational process for involving personnel in planning and executing a continuous stream of improvement in systems in order to provide quality health care that meets or exceeds customer expectations.

common cause variation. the inherent variability in a defined and controlled process after special cause variation has been corrected.

craft. individual and independent workers producing work according to their own process choices, which generally are not well codified. This production system is very flexible, but can be very inefficient.

gross domestic product. the sum of all goods and services produced in the economy of a country.

mass customization. a process that adapts the product or service to the needs of the customer using highly standardized modules, which are supported and integrated by information systems and efficient delivery methods.

mass production. making standardized goods or services in high volumes with a stable, defined process involving division of labor, little worker autonomy, and tight process controls.

publicly-held. a firm whose stock is owned by individuals other than the management and the founders or their heirs.

segmentation. the division of a population into groups and classifications that are suitable for market and service delivery analysis in detail.

special cause variation. variability in output or outcome quality induced by external individuals and events, which are driving the process away from its natural distribution of outcomes.

underwriting. the analysis of an individual or group to determine whether or not to provide insurance coverage and, if so, to set the benefits to be provided at a given premium level or the price to be charged for a given level of benefits.

REFERENCES

Adams, W.W., & Herzlinger, R.E. (1993). *South Eye Institute*. Cambridge, MA: Publishing Division, Harvard Business School.

Baker, F., Sheldon, A.C., & McLaughlin, C.P. (1970). *Systems analysis and medical care.* Cambridge, MA: M.I.T. Press.

Boynton, A.C., Victor, B., & Pine, B.J., III (1993). New competitive strategies: challenges to organizations and information technology. *IBM Systems Journal, 32,* 40–64.

Bunker, J.P., Barnes, B.A., & Mosteller, F. (1979). *The costs, risks and benefits of surgery.* Princeton, NJ: Princeton University Press.

Coile, R.J., Jr. (1997). *The five stages of managed care: strategies for providers, hmos, and suppliers.* Chicago: Health Administration Press.

Deming, W.A. (1986). *Out of Crisis.* Cambridge, MA: M.I.T. Center for Advanced Engineering Study.

Ezzy, R., & Scott, W. (1995). *County Physical Therapy, Caribou, ME.* Chapel Hill, NC: Kenan-Flagler Business School, University of North Carolina.

Halverson, P.K., Kalzuny, A.D., & McLaughlin, C.P. (Eds.) (1998). *Managed care and public health.* Gaithersburg, MD: Aspen Publishers.

Herzlinger, R.E. (1997). *Market driven health care.* Reading, MA: Addison-Wesley Publishing Co.

Ilinitch, A.Y., & McLaughlin, C.P. (1998). Privatizing the mental health system in King County, WA. In P.K. Halverson, A.D. Kaluzny & C.P. McLaughlin (Eds.), *Managed care and public health* (pp. 301–319). Gaithersburg, MD: Aspen Publishers.

Kongstvedt, P.R. (1997). *Essentials of managed health care,* (2nd ed.) Gaithersburg, MD: Aspen Publishers.

Masalin, L. (1994). *Orton Hospital: Turnaround in a health care organization.* Chapel Hill, NC: Kenan-Flagler Business School, University of North Carolina.

Mayer, T.R., & Mayer, G.G. (1985). HMOs: origins and development. *New England Journal of Medicine, 312,* 590–594.

McLaughlin, C.P. (1995). Balancing collaboration and competition: The Kingsport, Tennessee Experience. *The Joint Commission Journal on Quality Improvement, 21,* 646–655.

McLaughlin, C.P. (1997). Management in practice—a case of risks and rewards. In K.A. Miller & E.K. Miller (Eds.), *Making sense of managed care. Vol. III: Operational issues and practical answers* (pp. 99–113). Tampa, FL: American College of Physician Executives.

McLaughlin, C.P. (1998a). Privatizing a community hospital in Rocky Mount, NC. In P.K. Halverson, A.D. Kaluzny, & C.P. McLaughlin (Eds.), *Managed care and public health* (pp. 261–275).

McLaughlin, C.P. (1998b). Rebuilding community and regional collaboration: The Kingsport, Tennessee Experience. *The Joint Commission Journal on Quality Improvement, 24,* 601–608.

McLaughlin, C.P., & Kaluzny, A.D. (1994). *Continuous Quality Improvement in Health Care: Theory, Implementation and Application.* Gaithersburg, MD: Aspen Publishers, Inc.

McLaughlin, C.P., & Kaluzny, A.D. (1997). Total quality management issues in managed care. *Journal of Health Care Finance, 24*(1), 10–16.

McLaughlin, C.P., & Kaluzny, A.D. (1998). Managed care: the challenge ahead. *OR/MS Today, 25*(1), 24–27.

McLaughlin, C.P., Pathman, D., & Konrad, T.R. (1997). Maintaining the practice network. *Health Care Management Review, 22*(4), 19–31.

McLaughlin, C.P., & Simpson, K.N. (1994). Holston Valley Hospital and Medical Center. In C.P. McLaughlin & A.D. Kaluzny (pp. 335–358).

McLaughlin, C.P., & Simpson, K.N. (1998). The new realities in health care technology assessment in U.S. institutions. *International Journal of Technology Management, Special Issue on Management of Technology in Health Care, 15,* 507–521.

McLaughlin, C.P., & Tillman, R. (1995). *Corning-Franklin Health Group (B).* Chapel Hill, NC: Kenan-Flagler Business School, University of North Carolina.

Office of Technology Assessment. (1980). *The implications of cost-effectiveness analysis of medical technology.* Washington, DC: OTA, Congress of the United States and *Background Paper #1: Methodological Issue and Literature Review.*

Phelps, C.E. (1997). *Health economics* (2nd ed.) Reading, MA: Addison-Wesley Education Publishers.

Portela, M.C. (1995). *A Markov model for the estimation of costs in the treatment of AIDS Patients*. Unpublished doctoral dissertation, Department of Health Policy and Administration, School of Public Health, University of North Carolina at Chapel Hill.

Shortell, S.M., Gillies, R.R., Anderson, D.A., Erickson, K.M., & Mitchell, J.M. (1996). *Remaking health care in America: Building organized delivery systems*. San Francisco, CA: Jossey-Bass, Publishers.

Starr, P. (1982). *The social transformation of American medicine*. New York: Basic Books.

Strauss, W., & Howe, N. (1991). *Generations: The history of America's future, 1584 to 2069*. New York: William Morrow & Co.

Weinstein, S.M., & Stason, W.B. (1977). Foundations of cost-effectiveness analysis for health and medical practices. *The New England Journal of Medicine, 296*, 716–721.

CHAPTER 4

Managing Organizational Design to Lead Change in Health Care Enterprises

Peter J. Dean

TABLE OF CONTENTS

EXECUTIVE SUMMARY

This chapter discusses the value of organizational design to physician leaders in an executive MBA program. Organizations are dynamic and complex social systems formed to accomplish goals. Organizational design is a field of study that focuses on the viewing of the organization as a system and how the framework of that system interfaces and influences the performance of the individual. Organizational design combines systems theory and qualitative and quantitative organizational analysis to help choose the best strategy for change with the understanding there is no one best design. However, an organizational designer attempts to bring about the best interface of the key factors in an organization. Factors considered in organizational design include the following: the people performing their jobs, the measurement of the performance, the processes that make up the tasks the people perform, the systems that comprise the processes, the arrangements of the hierarchy and reporting relationships that make up the formal structure, the informal structure professionals create for themselves, and how the strategy of the organization aligns itself to all the aforementioned factors (Miles & Snow, 1978; Nadler, Gerstein, & Shaw, 1992). These factors are underpinned by the following organizational behaviors of managers: recognition of individual differences in workers, accurate perception of performance, correct assumptions about the motivation of workers, the information technology of organizational communication, the influence of conflict and collaboration on both group and team dynamics (Bowditch & Buono, 1997), and the management of operations as discussed in Chuck Noon's chapter.

In addition, organizational design involves developing a process to support both organizational learning and individual learning (Dean & Ripley, 1997; Drucker, 1993; Garvin, 1993; Senge, 1990; Watkins & Marsick, 1993). The process described in this chapter presents the design of the organization from becoming stagnant and allows the organization to shift its design to meet the demands of a changing business environment. Although this process is dynamic, there are some principles that stand firm and upon which a physician leader can build an organization that lasts. These principles central to organizational design are interpersonal communication, equity, fairness, free speech, teamwork, learning, and relearning. The knowledge of organizational design is essential for physician leaders who desire to positively influence health care enterprises.

INTRODUCTION

Global Change

The challenges of change in business today are global in scale. They range from sophisticated global competition and cooperation and demands for improved quality to the pressure to reduce the time it takes to communicate, produce, deliver, and respond to cost-cutting and downsizing agendas. These are among the realities of today's business. These and other sociopolitical and economic forces drive the need for change in organizations. The swift and demanding currents of change exist in health care as well. Health care organizations and hospitals are not inevitable institutions. They, too, are constantly negotiated and renegotiated in response to immediate crisis and the practicalities of change (Stevens, 1991).

Change in Health Care

Change in health care, reviewed more thoroughly in Chapter 1 by Curtis McLaughlin, includes a series of changes. At one time, such change was the shifting of financial risk from the 1950s to today.

The traditional fee-for-service transaction allowed health care professionals to provide services, and the patients paid as much of the fees for these services as they could. The fee-for-service transaction changed over the 1960s and 1970s when the federal government and employers began to pay for health care coverage. As employers began to increase the amount of health care benefits, they began to forecast how much money should be set aside for future health care bills. Designing the organization around these changes challenged health care leaders. Insurance companies responded to this need by offering indemnity policies to employers. The insurance policies were set up so the employer paid a fixed fee to an insurance company, the health care professional provided services, and the insurance company paid usual and customary fees for services.

Employers were willing to prepay a fixed fee to an insurance company to limit their financial responsibility. The insurance company assumed all of the risk associated with the health care bills of those employees for that year. The fee charged by the insurance company was typically calculated by taking last year's costs and adding a profit margin. In this situation, the physician was paid directly by insurance companies and not the patient. If the insurance company experienced rising costs, the premium of the following year's insurance would go up. The design of this system had cascading effects and may have affected patient care in an adverse way, increasing the cost of health care to the people. Also, new technologies contributed to the rising costs of health care. In response to these rising costs, a new way to manage costs emerged in the marketplace—Managed Care. There was an even greater challenge for those designing organizations and trying to balance patient care and profitability. Managed care made it difficult to focus the design of organization systems totally centered on the patient care.

Managed care allows the employer to pay a fixed fee to a managed care company, the health care professional to provide services at a discount, the patient to pay a co-pay or deductible, and the managed care company to pay remaining fees for services.

Managed care is defined as a way of providing health care services within a defined network of health care providers who are given more responsibility to manage and provide quality, cost-effective care. In the early years of managed care, there existed a slowing down of health care costs. With evolution of health care plans and with employers becoming more demanding, the creators of health care plans had to better design ways of eliminating the unnecessary and redundant services. This resulted in a consequence where physicians had to think twice about which services to provide in each patient interaction. It is possible that by moving from Managed Care to full-risk contracts, the physician will have more control over how medicine is practiced.

Full-risk transactions consist of the following: the employer pays a fixed fee to the managed care company; the managed care company pays a fixed fee to a health system; the health care professional provides services; and the health system pays salary or capped fee to health care personnel.

These changes and the other changes in health care, listed by McLaughlin in Chapter 3, require a rethinking, redesigning, and restructuring of the health care enterprises that provide patient care. For this reason, it is important for physician leaders to have knowledge about the field of organizational design.

Organizational Design Helps Enterprises Adapt To Change

This chapter is about understanding and leading organizational design when dealing with change (Bennis, Benne, & Chin, 1985) in health care.

Information about organizational design helps a physician leader use discretion in the design of organizational factors, such as strategies, policies, structures, processes, systems, and tactics.

Organizational design (Argyris, 1993; Bowman & Kogut, 1995; Galbraith, 1977, 1995; Galbraith & Lawler, 1993) has become even more critical than it has always been for health care. Whether it is a multinational corporation, small business, hospital, HMO, government agency, or religious organization, the design of the organization matters in the overall organizational performance as well as the performance of the individuals. What kind of a shift is needed for an organization to achieve faster innovation and flexibility and to become a learning organization (Senge, 1990) as well as to achieve improved organizational and individual performance (Dean,1999)? The shift must move from the traditional, closed organization system with a rigid hierarchical structure that stresses centralized control and fixed boundaries to a more open, flexible hierarchy with a participative learning system (M. Emery, 1993). It is in this kind of organization where physician leaders and health care professionals foster two-way communication, decentralized decision making, informal networks cross-cutting formal boundaries, reciprocal information sharing, shared commitment to sustained cooperation and involvement, and a common set of values (Kochan & Useem, 1992). All of these features should be housed within a self-designing learning organization (Mohrman & Cummings, 1989).

ORGANIZATION DESIGN—WHAT HAS BEEN LEARNED

The following description of organizational design and its influence on individual performance was mostly drawn from Dean (1999), Robey and Sales (1994), Nadler and Tushman (1997), and Dean and Ripley (1997, 1998a, 1998b, 1998c). Organizational design involves the total system of formal arrangements housing the interaction of the structure, processes, and systems for the purpose of optimal learning. This total system interfaces between humans and the work the enterprise sets out to accomplish. The design of these arrangements can either enhance or hinder accomplishment of the shared purposes of the enterprise. The organizational designer develops these arrangements in such a way as to lead to the alignment among the broad organizational factors of organization, process, and the behavior of the performer (Cummings & Worley, 1993; Gilbert, 1996; Levinson, 1972; Rummler, 1997; Rummler & Brache, 1990). Organizational design manifests through its operations. Charles Noon's chapter in this volume shows how the operations manager implements the operational design. Further, the design must include a subsystem of arrangements involving and impacting the immediate work environment, the job, and the health care provider.

The terms used when discussing organizational design are defined below (Miles & Snow, 1978; Nadler, Gerstein, & Shaw, 1992; Nadler & Tushman, 1997; Tushman, O'Reilley, & Nadler, 1989). *Strategic vision* reveals how the organization acts to survive in the marketplace (see Chapter 2). *Structure* arranges how tasks are divided and coordinated using specialization and integration as well as decentralization and centralization and formal patterns of relationships between groups and individuals. *Processes* are specifically defined and measured using a sequence of steps, activities, and methods to produce a specified goal, result, or consequence for meeting the need of a particular internal/external customer or market. The different kinds of processes include the following: patient-care processes, task support processes, and information processes. *Systems* include all the procedures for budgeting, accounting, and training that make the organization run using a particular set of procedures/rules, policies, devices, guides, and practices that are designed to control processes in a predictable way. Examples from a staffing system might include the following:

- patient application forms
- patient reference checks
- patient exit interviews
- procedure for posting jobs
- applying for a transfer, and so on.

Cooperative learning of physician leaders and health care professionals requires working together for an integration of goals, policies, procedures, standards, information and feedback systems, incentive systems, training, and budget. Healthy alignment of these organizational factors in a balanced design brings about high-quality patient care and a competitive advantage (Utterback, 1994; von Bertalanffy, 1950, 1952; Weinberg, 1975).

Organizational design engages a physician leader to align functional groupings of the formal structures of the health care organization. This alignment requires asking such questions as the following:

- What departments report to what divisions?

- What is the degree of centralization and decentralization?
- What are the budget structures and procedures?
- How is decision-making authority set up?
- How are jobs designed?
- What are the control and coaching mechanisms for performance improvement?
- What is the role of human resource management systems?
- How does the physical location effect the ergonomics of work?

The processes and systems, or the sequence of tasks involved in implementing answers to these questions, must be consistently and flexibly arranged based on their value-added contributions to the health care organization. The explicit and implicit aspects of collaborative learning focus on the work itself. These aspects include the capacity, skill, and knowledge the worker must have, aligned with the provisions of the organization to inform, communicate, support, and recognize the worker's accomplishments. The opportunity to collaborate with fellow coworkers to improve their own performance also is important.

All the structures, systems and processes, and "learn-how" of the members of the organization, aligned with the strategy of the health care organization, must be considered as part and parcel of one connective system. Without learning and relearning, the system will become closed and unresponsive. Without continual process and systems redesign based on market demands, the system will not be connected with itself or the market demands. Without leadership the structure will not be designed in a way to compete effectively in the marketplace. Physician leaders who take on organization design in health care enterprise are taking on one of the most critical endeavors for the life cycle of the business in these rapidly changing times of the global market.

The "learn how" of an organization is crucial for good organizational design. According to de Geus (1997), enterprises die because managers focus only on the economic activity of producing goods or services and they forget that their organizations' true nature is that of a community of humans who are able to learn and adapt. A study performed in Royal Dutch/Shell Group (de Geus, 1997) found that the ability to return investment to shareholders seemed to have little to do with longevity. Profits were necessary for short-term cash flow and to focus the company, but were not a predictor or determinant of corporate health. De Geus (1997) suggested that profits were a symptom of health and not the root cause.

He suggested that the root cause was the company's ability to grasp the need for change and adapt to it. De Geus went on to suggest that a key for survival was an organization's tolerance for learning. That translates into giving employees a certain amount of freedom and space to improve the business operations without fear of reprisal. This suggests people should be free to improve on the efficiency of tasks. In addition, the organization is designed so that learning can be disseminated quickly and occur going up, down, and laterally across the functions of an enterprise.

How To Avoid Inflexibility and Optimize Organizational Design

Inflexibility in organizational design brings about rigid assumptions about power and risk avoidance in communication. These are old habits that will not work anymore. Hammer and Champy (1993) suggested that this inflexibility comes from the fragmentation of the workforce through specialization, rigid hierarchy, and the control of work not being in the hands of the workers. To deal with the inflexibility of these organizations, Kochan and Useem (1992) suggested continuous, systemic organizational change that is integrated and consistent among an organization's major components and long-term orientation to provide a more suitable foundation for cooperation, learning, and innovation. Galbraith and Lawler (1993) stated that organizations would need to design themselves through innovation and process improvement. They went on to suggest that the successful organizations would be those that can better design their organization to meet the new realities of business. Kochan and Useem (1992) suggested that learning and learning how to learn are the essential capacities for an organization to better design itself. Gilbert (1996) and Dean (1999, in press) suggest that organizational design emerge from individuals operating from different levels of vantage within an organization. These are the different contexts in which one could look at what happens with the organization and, therefore, subsequent changes to design occurring from these vantage points would be more effective. They include the following:

- Philosophical: the ideals under which the organization operates.
- Cultural: the larger environment in which the organization exists.
- Policy: the vision and missions that define the purpose of the organization.
- Strategic: the plans designed to carry out the mission.
- Tactical: the specific duties that achieve the strategies.

- Logistical: the support system (resources, information, incentives, etc.) that enables workers to carry out duties.

Whatever the suggestions for design and change from the many vantage points of an organization might be, one idea begins to become more clear and loom large as a critical need.

Organizational Design Decisions Directly Impact Performance

Attempts at organizational design are often limited. Why? Failure often results from a phenomenon that exists as a fundamental attribution error in everyday inferences about cause–effect relations, according to Jitendra Vir Singh (1998, personal communication) of The Wharton School, The University of Pennsylvania.

The fundamental attribution error predisposes individuals to overemphasize humans as the cause of the problem and underestimate the role environmental factors play in causing resistance to plans for change. This results in managerial decision makers trying not to influence behavior in the workplace by designing organization contexts but by trying to fix the individuals in the workplace. In the past, performance was perceived as separate from the environment within which the performance occurred. There was no concept that how the direction of the company was framed or structured could impact the work and the people. Far less was the idea that the work environment could be a source of revival, renewal, and re-creation of energy. As Singh (1998) suggested above, organizational design decisions directly impact the performance of work. Organizational design, utilizing a performance improvement mental model (Dean & Ripley, 1997), speaks to the total system within which physician leaders make decisions about the configuration or architecture of the design factors in the formal organization including the formal structures, processes, and systems. This sets the tone for how the work gets done, the way the people perform their job, and the morale of the workplace. For example, a physician leader would work with the distribution of information processes, such as an electronic performance support system (Dean & Ripley, 1997), to do the following:

- Effectively communicate expectations.
- Continuously feedback the results of performance.
- Objectively allocate resources for task support such as tools, materials, equipment, supplies and, especially, time to do the work.

- Consistently base the rewards, recognition, and incentives on the actual work performed.

The decisions about the design of an organization have direct bearing on the individual performance. Knowledge of performance improvement models, methods, and measures (Dean & Ripley, 1997, 1998a, 1998b, 1998c) can be useful for the diffusion of the design within the organization.

A Physician Can Lead Change with Organizational Design

The real test of leadership in business that allows a company to age for a longer time and avoid premature expiration of a business life cycle seems to be the ongoing achievement of two kinds of change. Increasing alignment among the strategy, structure, process, people, and learning through incremental or evolutionary change marks long-term success. This incremental change is punctuated by discontinuous or radical change that requires the simultaneous shift in strategy, structure, process, people, and learning (Tushman & O'Reilly, 1996). Cost-containment, efficiency, and incremental innovation mark continuous change. Organizational performance problems, or technological, competitive shifts in the market, regulatory events, or political conditions almost always drive discontinuous change. Speed, flexibility, and radical innovations are critical to adaptation in crises. Almost all successful organizations go through periods of incremental change punctuated by discontinuous or radical change. This can be caused by the following:

- Deregulation such as in the financial and airline industries led to waves of mergers and failures as companies worked frantically to redesign themselves.
- Political change such as in Eastern Europe and South Africa has had a similar impact as firms reorient themselves to the radical pressure for change.
- Technological change such as in the microprocessor industry revolutionized the computer industry.

TWO KINDS OF CHANGE IN ORGANIZATIONS

Although not an example from health care, the story of Apple Computer (Tushman and O'Reilly, 1996) illustrates the two kinds of change an organization experiences. The history of Apple Computer begins with a small group of individuals designing, producing, and selling a personal computer. That was not the only reason for their success. The design of their organization had a high degree of alignment and congruence among the strategy of the organization and their organizational design (structure, systems of design, manufacturing, marketing, distribution, and accounting/payroll, processes of critical tasks needed to implement the systems). People had assigned roles and a learning culture based on shared values of innovation, commitment, and speed.

With success and growth several changes began to happen. Apple got larger and needed a different design, so more structure, systems, and processes were added for efficiency and control. The learning culture changed to reflect new challenges as new norms emerged to show what was important and what would not be tolerated. This slowed creativity, and the joy of learning staled conversation about all the potential possibilities. This slowing of creative ventures was due to energy being put into the new learning that had to occur for continued success and it depended on using what worked and eliminating what did not work.

In addition, Apple's strategy changed from a single product for personal computer users with a focused strategy to a broader range of products with a market-wide emphasis on user, educational institutions, and industrial markets. For Apple to ensure congruence and alignment of its organizational design and its people, and with this evolved strategy based on changing markets and technology, new leadership was brought into the company. Steve Jobs was out and John Sculley was in.

Other things required change as well. As the product type matured, the basis of competition changed. Early on, competition was based on product variation, whereas later on it shifted to features, efficiency, and cost. When Mac, IBM's OS/2, and Microsoft Windows competed with each other, it was based on product variation, until Windows became industry standard in operating systems. Then competition shifted to cost, quality, and efficiency. This required changes in the design of the organization, as Apple had to once again redesign the congruence among strategy, organizational design (the structure, systems, and processes), the people, and the culture. Now, Sculley was "out" and Spindler was " in" to move operations into a more mature market. With organizational performance at a standstill, Apple's Board of Directors chose Gil Amelio to turn it around.

Over a 20-year period, Apple's incremental change was punctuated by discontinuous change. Each of these different periods in Apple's history required radical changes in the design of structures, systems, processes, people and learning, and leadership skills so that the new strategy would be in alignment with the new design. The take-away from these experiences in business is that eventually, alignment or congruence of a successful firm, or even an industry will be upset by discontinuities. Perhaps the health care industry is in need of more than incremental change. Whether one agrees with this point or not, there are some guidelines one can follow in using the knowledge of organizational design when dealing with change.

AN ORGANIZATIONAL DESIGN PROCESS

Hupp (1998) developed a process for designing work to achieve fit among purpose or strategy, processes, and people. The organization by design process (Hupp, 1998), as described below, was created from the following selected sources: Galbraith (1977, 1995), Trist (1981), Weisbord (1987, 1992), Cummings and Worley (1993), M. Emery (1993), and Bunker and Alban (1997). It is important to remember that the purpose is not to create the perfect design, but to create a design of a self-adaptive system. The three parts of this overall, self-adaptive system include the following:

1. Environment (the external context) interacting with the strategic direction (the organization's response, its corresponding purpose, and strategy). This captures the need of the physician leaders for the knowledge of organizational design. The categories of this knowledge are environmental pressures of international business on the organization; flexibility of the organization's structure and its design; knowing the uniqueness of the organization's culture and potential competing values; know-how and learn-how of managing large-scale organizational change supported by appropriate developmental techniques; and understanding group dynamics and group process during change, especially in relationship to conflict and collaboration.

2. Work process and technology involve the work processes and tools that it takes to produce the organization's products and services, how the information flows, and the measure of the accomplishment of work. This captures the need of alignment in organizational design factors discussed above. The knowledge that enables a physician leader to bring about this change involves understanding the

interactions among power, leadership, and management; understanding the importance of information technology (see chapters by Jackson and Ray in this volume); and understanding the importance of comprehensive organizational communication and interpersonal communication.

3. People, their performance, their organizational structures, and HR systems involve how people are organized, how authority and responsibility are distributed, how people are selected, developed, and rewarded. This ensures that the focus is on the professionals practicing patient care. What enables a physician leader for this part includes the following: understanding how people are different in their work styles; understanding how people perceive differently owing to their positions; understanding how a worker's attitude is actually shaped by his or her style and perception; understanding how the motives of people are impacted by their attitude and by the feedback they receive from the work environment.

Self-Designing System Concept

A self-designing system (Hupp, 1998) is designed to do the following:

1. Be increasingly self-regulating and more responsive to its business context.
2. Deploy a work process that is fast, focused, and flexible.
3. Include members with the collective expertise to plan, coordinate, control, and troubleshoot their own start-to-finish work process.
4. Construct jobs that build contributors' ownership and commitment.

Key design principles for a self-designing system drawn from the literature of organizational design summed up by Hupp (1998) include the following:

- Think in Wholes

  1. The best design for a productive system is one in which each part of the system embodies the goals of the overall system. Maintain principles of ethics as standards (see the chapter by Dean and Massingale in this volume) against which to measure true progress (Argyris, 1982; Argyris & Schon, 1980; Emery, 1969; Ghoshal & Barlett, 1997).

2. Joint optimization: Effectiveness of the whole is more important than effectiveness of the parts.

- Create Self-Regulating Units

    1. Units should be sufficiently self-regulating so that they can cope with problems and seize opportunities by rearranging their own resources (F.E. Emery, 1995; Emery & Trist, 1960, 1973; Emery & Purser, 1996; M. Emery, 1993; Trist, 1981).
    2. Provide internal coordination and control. Provide information and discretion directly to those who need it, when they need it.
    3. Provide requisite variety in control systems. Internal flexibility should be appropriate to environmental variability. Feedback systems should be as complex as the variances they need to control.
    4. Provide for redundancy of functions (multiskilled contributors) rather than redundancy of parts (staffing to support narrowly sliced, specialized functions). Enhance capacity by enlarging roles, not by adding specialists.
    5. The design process should set "minimal critical specifications." Do not carve in stone what should be left to local discretion.

- View People As a Resource with Free Speech, Not As a Commodity

    1. Provide jobs that meet M. Emery's (1993) six psychological criteria:
    —Elbow room (autonomy)
    —Learning (allow individuals to set goals and get direct feedback)
    —Variety
    —Mutual support and respect
    —Meaningfulness (allow doers to "see the big picture" and create something important)
    —A desirable future

- Walk the Talk—"Be the Change You Want To See"

    1. Use a change process that demonstrates and reinforces the outcomes you hope to achieve.
    2. The design process is more about getting the system to see and adapt itself than it is about perfecting workflow and structure. Redesign should be participative, not representative. That is, redesign should be done by people who must make the redesign work, not by a representative design team in isolation.

Realize that it is never finished. You are not making a transition between one stable state and another. You are moving from one period of transition to another.

There are unique benefits of large-scale organizational design conferences by the stakeholders (Hupp, 1998). When you design work to align strategic direction, work processes, organizational structure, and jobs, you can get the following:

- Better coordination and information flow. When you organize work around whole products or services, people who need to cooperate with each other are on the same team, focused on a common goal. (In the past, work has typically been organized around functions, putting people who need to cooperate with each other on different work groups, pursuing function-specific goals.)
- Reduced costs and cycle time. When you streamline workflow, you remove or minimize non-value-adding steps. This reduces cost, cycle time, and opportunity for error. In addition, when mature work teams plan and monitor their own work, you need fewer managers. The managers who remain can focus on integrating efforts across teams and developing business strategy.
- Improved responsiveness to customers. When you organize work around products, services, or customer groups, employees get greater access to customers, become better at anticipating customer needs, and provide better informed, more responsive customer service.
- More innovation. When you provide employees with the opportunity and responsibility to improve their products, services, and processes, you shorten the distance between ideas and their implementation.
- More value added through people. When employees produce whole products or services, not isolated fragments, they take more ownership over their jobs. Also, jobs that integrate thinking with doing result in greater job satisfaction. Finally, when managers focus on integrating, instead of supervising, they concentrate on getting people to work together across boundaries, not second-guessing individual efforts. This focuses them on adding value, not reworking their subordinates' work.
- More flexibility. When the organization deploys a broadly skilled work force it gets more flexibility than when it deploys a narrowly skilled one.

Hupp (1998) recommended some special precautions for large-scale organizational design:

- Management needs to do the hard work of thinking through what it will and will not accept on the front end.
- Aligning the organization (becoming an open, learning system where the workers who perform the core process are invested with the authority and accountability to plan, make decisions, and seize opportunities that are embedded in their processes) involves a fundamental power shift from the following:

  1. Hierarchical to participative power.
  2. Expert diagnosis and prescription (doing it *to* the line organization) to line contributors examining and adapting their own system (doing it *through* the line organization).

Before you begin the process, confirm that management is ready for this shift. Make sure it intends to become strategic rather than tactical, integrative rather than empire-building, resource brokering rather than resource controlling. Members of the planning or steering team need to play the role of advocates, not critics, of the process. Change management means more than good public relations. It means engaging stakeholders in working through the real conflicts and polarities that underlie differences, not smoothing them over with sound bites.

If you use large-scale conferencing methodologies (Bunker & Alban, 1997; Cabana, 1995; Dean, 1983, 1993; Dean, Dean, & Guman, 1992), facilitators need to make sure that the conferences allow enough time and provide forums to engage the real conflict and polarities that exist in the system. Facilitators need to be skilled in building sustainable agreements among diverse stakeholders. Sponsors, advocates, and consultants need to remember that the ultimate answers are not in the methodology—it is simply a tool. The system's stakeholders already have all the wisdom they need to find their answers. It's the job of sponsors, advocates, and consultants to get them to discuss the right questions, so they can collectively uncover the truth that is already there, buried under organizational clutter.

CONCLUSION

Leadership of an organization emerges when the company is able to compete successfully by continuously aligning strategy, structure, and processes, and learning to deal with the needs of incremental change while simultaneously preparing for radical change caused by the discontinuous pressure of the external market. This requires that the organization be designed to account for competition in a mature market where cost, efficiency, and incremental innovation are vital while developing new products and services where speed, flexibility, and radical change are critically important (Lawrence & Lorsch, 1967, 1969; Tushman & O'Reilly, 1996). Both of these notions are easily understood, yet usurping one to make more sumptuous the other may create short-term success but will eventually lead the organization to long-term failure. Leading organizations proactively align their strategy, structure, processes, people, and culture through incremental evolutionary change. This change is punctuated by radical and discontinuous change that requires simultaneous shifting of the strategy, structure, processes, people, and culture to deal with sudden changes in technology, regulatory events, changes in the political environment, economic conditions, and competitive shifts in the market (Tushman & O'Reilly, 1996). It is the knowledge of some kind of organizational design process, maybe even a self-designing process, that is required by management to deal with this phenomenon (Axelrod, 1992; Beckhard, 1969; Beckhard & Harris, 1987; Bunker & Alban, 1997; Lewin, 1945, 1947a, 1947b, 1948, 1951; Likert, 1961, 1967; Lippitt, 1967, 1980, 1983; Weisbord, 1987, 1992; Weisbord & Janoff, 1995; McLagan & Christo, 1995).

All of a physician leader's decisions to deal with organizational design depend upon the performers in the organization and the process they are allowed to use, enabling them to deal with both kinds of change, incremental and discontinuous. If leaders try to adapt to discontinuities through incremental adjustments, they are not likely to succeed. If leaders try to do it alone, they are not likely to succeed. If you influence the design of the organizational system, you influence that system, which has a direct influence over individual performer. For those using systems thinking for the entire organization, they are dealing with performance improvement endeavors, which we call organizational designers. Organizational design helps companies organize themselves and deal with the complexities of organizational life. In health care, the physician leader must have knowledge of organizational design to lead the changing destiny of health care in this country.

GLOSSARY

continuous change. learning that occurs in an incremental way usually motivated by cost-containment, efficiency, and evolutionary innovation.

cooperative learning. workers learning and helping each other learn for a specific outcome.

discontinuous change. learning that occurs in a radical way driven by performance or technological problems, competitive shifts in the market, or political conditions.

learning organization. an organization where cooperative and reflective learning occurs in response to the needs of the organization, thus helping the organization become self-designing.

organizational design. the total system of formal arrangements in an organization encompassing the interaction of the strategy, structures, processes, and systems. These arrangements are designed in such a way to optimize the learning interface between people and their work environment.

performance. both behavior, the actual observable activity, and its accomplishment, that which is left behind after the behavior occurs, define performance. That is, behavior plus accomplishment equal performance.

processes. processes define and measure the sequence of steps, activities, and methods to produce a specific goal or outcome.

strategic vision. the response of the organization to the needs of the marketplace.

structures. structure addresses the division and coordination of tasks and the formal patterns of relationships between groups and individuals.

systems. systems include all the procedures for budgeting, accounting, training, and so on that make the organization run. Systems use procedures, rules, policies, practices, and so on that help control processes.

REFERENCES

Argyris, C. (1982). *Reasoning, learning, and action: individual and organizational.* San Francisco, CA: Jossey-Bass, Publishers.

Argyris, C. (1993). *Knowledge for action: A guide to overcoming barriers to organizational change.* San Francisco, CA: Jossey-Bass, Publishers.

Argyris, C., & Schon, D.A. (1980). *Organizational learning: A theory of action perspective.* Reading, MA: Addison-Wesley Publishing Co.

Axelrod, D. (1992). Getting everyone involved: How one organization involved its employees, supervisors and managers in redesigning the organization. *Journal of Applied Behavioral Science, 28,* 499–509.

Beckhard, R. (1969). *Organization development: Strategies and models.* Cambridge, MA: MIT Press.

Beckhard, R., & Harris, R. (1987). *Organizational transitions: Managing complex change* (2nd ed.). Reading, MA: Addison-Wesley Publishing Co.

Bennis, W.G., Benne, K.D., & Chin, R. (1985). *The planning for change.* New York: Holt, Rinehart and Winston.

Bowditch, J.L., & Buono, A.F. (1997). *A primer on organizational behavior.* New York: John Wiley & Sons.

Bowman, E., & Kogut, B. (1995). *Redesigning the firm.* New York: Oxford University Press.

Bunker, B.B., & Alban, B.T. (Eds.). (1997). *Large group interventions: Engaging the whole system for rapid change.* San Francisco: Jossey-Bass, Publishers.

Cabana, S. (1995). Participative design works, partially participative doesn't. *Journal for Quality and Participation, 18,* 10–19.

Cummings, T.G., & Worley, C.G. (1993). *Organization development and change.* St. Paul, MN: West Publishing Co.

Dean, P.J. (1983). *Guidelines for the implementation of change by a change team.* Unpublished manuscript, The University of Iowa, Iowa City.

Dean, P.J. (1993). *Re-engineering the business enterprise by organizational redesign.* Unpublished manuscript, The Penn State University, Great Valley, PA.

Dean, P.J. (1995). Examining the practice of human performance technology. *Performance Improvement Quarterly, 8,* 68–94.

Dean, P.J. (1999). *Performance engineering at work* (2nd ed.). Washington, DC: International Society for Performance Improvement and the International Board of Standards for Training, Performance and Instruction.

Dean, P.J., Dean, M.R., & Guman, E. (1992). Identifying a range of performance improvement solutions—high yield training to systems redesign. *Performance Improvement Quarterly, 5*(4), 16–32.

Dean, P.J., & Ripley, D.E. (1997). *Performance improvement pathfinders: Models for organizational learning systems.* Washington, DC: International Society for Performance Improvement Publications.

Dean, P.J., & Ripley, D.E. (Eds.). (1998a). Performance improvement interventions: Methods for organizational learning: Instructional design and training (Vol. 2). Washington, DC: International Society of Performance Improvement.

Dean, P.J., & Ripley, D.E. (Eds.). (1998b). Performance improvement interventions: Methods for organizational learning: Performance technologies in the workplace (Vol. 3). Washington, DC: International Society of Performance Improvement.

Dean, P.J., & Ripley, D.E. (Eds.). (1998c). Performance improvement interventions: Methods for organizational learning: Culture and systems change (Vol. 4). Washington, DC: International Society of Performance Improvement.

de Geus, A. (1997). *The living company: Habits for survival in a turbulent business environment.* Cambridge, MA: Harvard Business School.

Drucker, P.F. (1993). *The ecological vision: Reflections on the American condition.* New Brunswick, NJ: Transaction Publishers.

Emery, F.E. (Ed.). (1969). *Systems thinking.* New York: Penguin.

Emery, F.E. (1978). *Systems thinking.* New York: Penguin.

Emery, F.E. (1995). Participative design: Effective, flexible and successful, now! *Journal for Quality and Participation, 18,* 6–9.

Emery, F.E., & Trist, E.L. (1960). Socio-technical systems. In C. W. Churchman & M. Verhulst (Eds.), *Management sciences, models and techniques* (pp. XX–XX). Tarrytown, NY: Pergamon.

Emery, F.E., & Trist, E.L. (1973). *Toward a social ecology.* New York: Plenum Publishing.

Emery, M. (Ed.) (1993). *Participative design for participative democracy.* Unpublished manuscript, Center for Continuing Education, Australian National University.

Emery, M., & Purser, R.E. (1996). *The search conference: Theory and practice.* San Francisco, CA: Jossey-Bass, Publishers.

Galbraith, J.R. (1977). *Organization design.* Reading, MA: Addison-Wesley Publishing Co.

Galbraith, J.R. (1995). *Designing organizations.* San Francisco, CA: Jossey-Bass, Publishers.

Galbraith, J.R., & Lawler, E.D. (1993). *Organizing for the future.* San Francisco, CA: Jossey-Bass, Publishers.

Garvin, D.A. (1993). Building a learning organization. *Harvard Business Review. July–August,* 78–91.

Ghoshal, S., & Bartlett, C.A. (1997). *The individualized corporation.* New York: Harper Business.

Gilbert, T.F. (1996). *Human competence: Engineering worthy performance.* Washington, DC: International Society for Performance Improvement.

Hammer, M., & Champy, J. (1993). Reengineering the corporation: A Manifesto for business revolution. New York: Harper Business.

Hupp, T.R. (1998). *Personal correspondence with the president of Organizations By Design,* Warrenville, IL.

Kochan, T.A., & Useem, M. (1992). *Transforming organizations.* New York: Oxford University Press.

Lawrence, P.R., & Lorsch, J.W. (1967). *Organization and environment: Managing differentiation and integration.* Boston, MA: Division of Research, Harvard Business School

Lawrence, P.R., & Lorsch, J.W. (1969). *Developing organizations: Diagnosis and action.* Reading, MA: Addison-Wesley Publishing Co.

Levinson, H. (1972). *Organizational diagnosis.* Cambridge, MA: Harvard University Press.

Lewin, K. (1947a). Frontiers in group dynamics, part 1: Channels of group life: Social planning and action research. *Human Relations, 1,* 143–153.

Lewin, K. (1947b). Frontiers in group dynamics, part 1: Concept, method and reality in social science: Social Equilibria and social change. *Human Relations, 1,* 5–41.

Lewin, K. (1948). *Resolving social conflicts.* New York: Harper & Row.

Lewin, K. (1951). *Field theory in social science.* New York: HarperCollins Publishers.

Lewin, K., French, J.R.P., Jr., Lipitt, R., Hendry, C., Kuselewitz, D., Emerson Deets, L., Zander, A. (1945). The practicality of democracy. In G. Murphy (Ed.), *Human nature and enduring peace* (pp. 295–347). Boston: Houghton Mifflin.

Likert, R. (1961). *New patterns of management.* New York: McGraw-Hill.

Likert, R. (1967). *The human organization.* New York: McGraw-Hill.

Lippitt, R. (1967). *Utilization of scientific knowledge for change in education. Concepts for social change.* Washington, DC: NTL Laboratories.

Lippitt, R. (1980). *Choosing the future you prefer.* Washington, DC: Development Publishers.

Lippitt, R. (1983). Future before you plan. In R.A. Ritvo & A.G. Sargent (Eds.), *The NTL managers' handbook* (pp. XX–XX). Arlington, VA: NTL Institute.

McLagan, P., & Christo, N. (1995). *The age of participation.* San Francisco, CA: Berrett-Koehler.

Miles, R.E., & Snow, C.C. (1978). *Organizational strategy, structure and process.* New York: McGraw-Hill.

Mohrman, S.A., & Cummings, T.G. (1989). *Self-designing organizations: Learning how to create high performance.* New York: Addison-Wesley Publishing Co.

Nadler, D.A., Gerstein, M.S., & Shaw, R.B. (1992). *Organizational architecture: Designs for changing organizations.* San Francisco, CA: Jossey-Bass, Publishers.

Nadler, D.A., & Tushman, M.L. (1997). *Competing by design: The power of organizational architecture.* New York: Oxford University Press.

Robey, D., & Sales, C.A. (1994). *Designing organizations.* Burr Ridge, IL: Irwin.

Rummler, G.A. (1997). Managing the organization as a system. *Training,* February, 68–74.

Rummler, G.A., & Brache, A.P. (1990). *Improving performance—How to manage the white space on the organization chart.* San Francisco, CA: Jossey-Bass, Publishers.

Senge, P.M. (1990). *The fifth discipline: The art and practice of the learning organization.* New York: Doubleday.

Stevens, R.A. (1991). The hospital as a social institution. *Hospital and Health Services Administration, 36,* 163–173.

Trist, E. (1981). The evolution of socio-technical systems: A conceptual framework and an action research program. *Occasional Paper* No.2. Philadelphia: University of Pennsylvania.

Tushman, M.L., & O'Reilly, C. (1996). Ambidextrous organizations: Managing evolutionary and revolutionary change. *California Management Review, 38*, 8–30.

Tushman, M.L., O'Reilly C., & Nadler, D.A. (1989). *The management of organizations: Strategies, tactics, analyses.* New York: Harper & Row.

Utterback, J. (1994). *Mastering the dynamics of innovation.* Boston, MA: HBS Press

von Bertalanffy, L. (1950). *General systems theory.* New York: George Braziller.

von Bertalanffy, L. (1952). *Problems of life.* New York: John Wiley & Sons.

Watkins, K.E., & Marsick, V.J. (1993). *Sculpting the learning organization: Lessons in the art and science of systemic change.* San Francisco, CA: Jossey-Bass, Publishers.

Weinberg, G.M. (1975). *An introduction to general systems thinking.* New York: John Wiley & Sons.

Weisbord, M.R. (1987). *Productive workplaces: Organizing and managing for dignity, meaning, and community.* San Francisco, CA: Jossey-Bass, Publishers.

Weisbord, M.R. (1992). *Discovering common ground.* San Francisco, CA: Berrett-Koehler.

Weisbord, M.R., & Janoff, S. (1995). *Future search.* San Francisco, CA: Berrett-Koehler.

CHAPTER 5

The Practice of Marketing: What Every Physician Leader Needs To Know

Sarah Fisher Gardial

TABLE OF CONTENTS

EXECUTIVE SUMMARY

For many physician leaders, the need to understand and practice marketing might well be considered a necessary evil: necessary due to the changing, competitive nature of the health care industry, and evil because it is often misperceived as a distasteful, unprofessional, and potentially manipulative aspect of business. Health care is, indeed, becoming increasingly competitive, and marketing efforts are often an appropriate response in such an environment. In addition, here are other compelling environmental reasons why health care providers should adopt a marketing focus, including a more demanding and sophisticated patient population and the challenge of responding to multiple, competing customer groups. Despite these trends, many misperceptions exist, which hamper physicians' desire to more enthusiastically embrace a marketing orientation. Most of these consist of biases and misunderstandings that are easily debunked by a clearer understanding of the Marketing Concept, the cornerstone philosophy of marketers. In addition, executive MBA programs should concentrate on helping physician leaders gain strategic focus through Market Opportunity Analysis (MOA) and Customer Value Determination (CVD). These fundamental frameworks provide a unifying orientation for the many marketing strategy decisions that are made by health care organizations, including new product development, promotion and communications, market segmentation and targeting strategies, health care delivery and access options, customer satisfaction measurement, and personnel/staff training. Through better understanding of these key marketing topics, physician leaders will find that they have both a valuable and indispensable perspective for responding to their changing world.

THE ENVIRONMENTAL IMPERATIVE: WHY PHYSICIANS NEED TO EMBRACE MARKETING

The health care profession, which was once considered "a calling" and the "art of healing," is now being discussed and managed using terms such as "markets," "cost controls," "revenue producing programs," "total quality management," and "financial returns." Whether one feels that the pendulum has swung too far toward these "bottom line" issues or not, the unavoidable conclusion is that the management and delivery of health care is now considered, fundamentally, a business that can never completely return to its former cottage industry approach (see Chapter 3,

"Health Policy for Physician Leaders"). For this reason, many physicians are attempting to arm themselves with additional business acumen to influence, participate in, and survive within the changing environment. My experience is that many physicians are eager to learn about the "financial" as well as the "management" concerns relevant to organizing and running an efficient and effective operation (topics which are unquestionably important). On the other hand, there is much more ambivalence regarding the topic of marketing.

However, there are plenty of legitimate and pressing reasons why marketing, as a general orientation, and marketing skills, specifically, are desirable tools in today's management and delivery of health care. Three of these key factors include the following: (1) increasing competition among health care players, (2) changing customer/patient attitudes, and (3) the multiple, competing customer groups that physicians must now serve. Each of these will be briefly discussed below.

Increasing Competition

Marketing emerged as a serious business discipline in the United States during the period following World War II (Hansen, 1977). At that time, resources that had been focused on the war effort turned inward, resulting in industrial productivity, the proliferation of new products and services, a booming economy, and an industrial complex stoked to feed a growing and more affluent population. In turn, this encouraged competition among suppliers who had to fight for market share, had to vie for customer loyalty, and could no longer assure longevity simply through greater productivity. In such a world, it was imperative to provide products that were more closely matched to the needs of the customer base and were superior to competitor offerings.

It was precisely at this time that the "Marketing Concept" emerged as a way of bringing customer concerns more "front and center" in a company's strategic decisions. (This concept will be discussed more fully in a later section, "What Is Marketing?") Marketing as a discipline began to systematically study and identify ways for both understanding and responding to customer needs. In short, where organizations had historically been "internally focused" on production concerns, marketing became a way of better aligning a company's internal capabilities with its external market/customer demands.

For many years the health care industry in the United States enjoyed seemingly unbridled growth and opportunity as gauged by spending and cost data ("National health expenditures as a percent of GDP," 1997). More recently some have warned of a slowing of these trends, as well as oversupply in the industry ("Tracking health care costs: An update," 1997). These warnings were not well heard or heeded at a time when hospitals were fueling their balance sheets through asset growth (primarily bricks and mortar), medical schools continued to produce doctors in record numbers, and physician incomes continued to grow at a healthy clip. To some extent, this reversal of trends is due to the long-term shift in the balance of health care supply versus demand. However, this shift has also been compounded by recent consolidation of health care deliverers and insurers, resulting in increasing power and clout among larger players. As health care providers have been forced to respond to larger, more powerful competitors in an oversupplied market, the issues of attracting and retaining customers have become more urgent. As with other industries before, marketing expertise has been ratcheted up to help health care organizations better understand and respond to customers in this increasingly competitive market. This is evidenced by the growing dollars devoted to health care marketing ("Hospitals boost marketing expenses by 25%," 1994; "See a doctor, get a toaster," 1997) as well as increasing attention to the structure and staffing of the marketing departments in many health care organizations. These trends have caused health care providers to more carefully consider what a marketing orientation is and how it can best be used in today's environment.

The Changing Patient Environment

It is not enough that the competitive environment has changed, but the patient environment has changed as well. To some extent, this might be a natural result of buyers' increasing clout in an oversupplied market. However, this also mirrors a larger societal trend: that is, customers across the board are growing more sophisticated, they have access to and are utilizing greater amounts of information to evaluate providers, and they are demanding higher quality in exchange for their dollars and loyalty. There is no question that patients, as consumers, feel more highly empowered as a group than in the past (Isaacs, Swartz, & Swartz, 1992; Herzlinger, 1997; "Opening doctors' ears," 1997). The very fact that Congress is considering a "Patient Bill of Rights" reflects the growing activism and vocalism of this consumer group.

In contrast to previous generations who looked on their doctors as un-questioned authorities and decision makers regarding health issues, to-day's patient/consumers are more likely to view their physicians as "team members" with whom health care decisions are jointly discussed, consid-ered, and made. In a world where patient/consumers spend more out-of-pocket dollars on "alternative" health care treatments, outside of the pur-veyance of their physician's (and insurer's) influence, than on "traditional" health care options, it is clear that patients increasingly feel able to take matters into their own hands. Indeed, one can argue that the migration of health care dollars toward "complimentary" health care options, such as vitamins and herbs, acupuncture, massage, homeopathy, and the like, is evidence of the failure of "traditional" medical providers to meet patients' health care needs (Herzlinger, 1997).

Finally, as patients have become more proactive, health care organiza-tions have become increasingly interested in understanding their levels of satisfaction with current offerings. Patient satisfaction surveys are not particularly new in this regard. What is new, however, are the ways in which these data are being utilized. Some of the latest trends (although quite controversial among many health care providers) are to make patient satisfaction survey data publicly available in order to facilitate better deci-sion making among patients and employers choosing health care pro-viders ("California group publishes ranking," 1997; "How good is your HMO?" 1997). Again, this trend mirrors the demand for and proliferation of data in other industries. Still, it speaks to the increasing voice of the pa-tient in the health care debate, as well as the increasing importance of patient responsiveness as a key to longevity in this industry.

Multiple, Competing Customers

Although patients represent one important group to which physicians must respond, they are by no means the only group. As the balance of power has shifted in the direction of third-party payers, physicians have been forced to respond to this second "customer group" and to be respon-sive to their changing demands. (Generally, business persons refer to product/service end users; e.g., patients, as "consumers." "Customers" typically refer to other organizations or individuals "downstream" in the value chain through which the provider must "sell" its services to reach its end users; for example, insurers, HMOs, hospitals, and health care sys-tems. For the remainder of this chapter, the term "customer" will be used to encompass both consumers and customers in the health care industry, unless otherwise specified.) Unfortunately, and frequently, physicians are faced with conflicting requirements from patients and third-party payers. Delivering desired value to one group often runs completely counter to the needs or desires of the other. And these are not the only two customer groups that physicians serve. Physicians are increasingly feeling the strain of responding to the families of patients, the larger community, and the various health care organizations in which they serve. With the acknowledgement of each additional "customer group" comes the responsibility of understanding its unique value requirements, as well as the need to strategically tradeoff or reconcile the needs of multiple groups for the good of the whole.

In sum, whereas there may be others, the above represent three key environmental factors that are placing increasing demands on health care providers to understand and strategically respond to their customers' value requirements, the fundamental tenant of the marketing discipline. Let us now consider more specifically what marketing has to offer in addressing these problems.

WHAT IS MARKETING?

Marketing's Bad Rap: Misperceptions, Biases, and Misinformation

Because marketing is a relatively recent orientation within the health care community, it is fraught with misperceptions that keep providers from fully embracing it. In this respect, it is helpful to start by debunking some of the more common misperceptions and, in essence, beginning to define marketing by stating what it is not.

Misperception #1: "Marketing Is Selling"

Probably one of the most common misperceptions is that marketing is selling. Not only is this an overly narrow perspective, but it is one that carries a great deal of negative baggage: "selling" is bad, manipulative, or even potentially unethical. In contrast, true marketing is about exactly the opposite. It is about striving to understand customers' needs so precisely that they are served better—that value is created for customers. The distinction between selling and marketing has been expressed in the following way:

> "Selling focuses on the needs of the seller; marketing on the needs of the buyer. Selling is preoccupied with the seller's need

to convert his product into cash; marketing with the idea of satisfying the needs of the customer (Levitt, 1960)."

In fact, it is marketing's goal to be so attuned to customers' needs, and so effective at responding to them, that, as Peter Drucker suggests, "selling becomes superfluous (Drucker, 1973)."

Misperception #2: "Marketing Is Advertising"

This myth probably exists because advertising is the most visible of all of the marketing efforts as far as the customer is concerned. Advertising does play an important informative and educational function, in addition to its persuasive role. Even so, it is only one in a variety of ways marketers communicate with their customers (also including publicity, face-to-face communications, sales and promotions). In turn, communications efforts are only one of four larger elements by which marketers respond to customers (the "marketing mix" includes promotional activities as well as decisions relative to the product/service offering, pricing, and distribution). More important, the marketing mix merely represents the "tools" that are used to respond to strategic decisions regarding market opportunity, customer segmentation and targeting, and positioning strategies. Therefore, advertising is only a small part of a much bigger, more complex strategic orientation. To say that marketing is only about advertising is comparable to saying that health care is only about surgery.

Misperception #3: "Marketing Is Unprofessional"

Individuals who believe that marketing is only about "selling" or "advertising" are also likely to believe that marketing is "below" the health care profession. Part of this "unprofessional" bias is, no doubt, rooted in tradition. In the past, the health care industry has not needed to aggressively practice marketing, and therefore some may not consider it necessary today. Unfortunately, many will cling to the familiar, "time honored" ways of managing health care, despite evidence to the contrary.

Others believe that health care should be "above" the coarseness and baseness of conducting business. It should be held to a "higher standard" of professionalism. The issue, of course, is not health care versus business, but how the two may coexist comfortably. As for those who would believe that all business is somehow "dirty," the point must be made that where ethics, integrity, and professionalism are concerned, there are business organizations that span the continuum, as well as health care providers. Any stereotypes in this respect are just that.

Misperception #4: "Marketing Is All Art and No Science"

Many have discounted marketing because it is the "art" side of business. In fact, it is true that good marketing relies to a great extent on creativity and right-brain thinking. It can rarely be reduced to formulas, statistics, and decision rules. However, what many do not realize is that good marketing represents creativity that is firmly rooted in data. Marketing is best understood as the meeting place for data and intuition, analysis and creativity, left- and right-brain thinking.

Another belief closely related to the "Marketing Is Art" misperception is that anybody can do it. If there is no "science" behind the discipline, then one's opinion is just as good as anyone else's. It might never occur to managers that they could be accountants or CFOs without adequate training, but in many organizations the marketing functions are conducted by people with little to no formal training in the discipline. Although this is not meant to diminish "on the job training" or an individual's experience and innate skills, the latter certainly does not substitute for formal training. As we will see later, the body of knowledge that is relevant to marketing decisions is large and complex. In this way, the "Marketing Is Art" misperception can have dangerous repercussions for organizations where this is the prevailing belief.

By addressing the preceding misperceptions, we begin to understand more accurately what marketing is. Let us further explore this issue by defining the Marketing Concept, the philosophical basis of marketing decisions and activities within a firm.

The Marketing Concept

Most marketing texts refer to the birth of a philosophy, now known as the "Marketing Concept," around the mid-1950s in corporate, not academic, America. Although stated and restated in various ways across the years, the Marketing Concept can be defined as follows: "The Marketing Concept holds that the key to achieving organizational goals consists in determining the needs and wants of target markets and delivering the desired satisfactions more effectively and efficiently than competitors (Kotler, 1994)."

In fact, a very close adaptation of this concept already exists for the health care industry. "The *health care marketing concept* is a health system's management orientation that accepts that the key task of the system is to determine the wants, needs, and values of a target market(s) and shape the system in such a manner to deliver the desired level of satisfaction (Cooper, 1994)."

While there are subtle differences between the two definitions, most marketers agree that there are three key assumptions underlying this orientation: (1) the need to understand customers, (2) the need to coordinate efforts within an organization, and (3) doing so in a way that is congruent with achieving an organization's ultimate goals.

Understanding Customer Needs

Understanding the needs of customers is the cornerstone of the marketing concept. In fact, marketers consider understanding and fulfilling customer needs to be the starting point for *all* strategic decisions within an organization. How to do so "effectively and efficiently" while "achieving organizational goals" are the parameters within which the creation and delivery of customer value occurs. It turns out that this seemingly intuitive and straightforward element of the marketing concept may be the most difficult to accomplish. In case after case, one can identify the cause of business failures to be organizations' inability to understand their customers' value requirements. Often, organizations move forward on decisions regarding product offerings, promotion, pricing, and the like without complete customer understanding (or worse still, with *mis*understanding). I actually believe that most organizations *want* to create value for their customers. Where they fall down is by not investing the time and effort it takes to truly understand their customers' often dynamic and changing requirements. This is "Job #1" for marketers. All of the strategic decisions that follow are simply matters of translating customer value requirements into action for the organization.

Coordinating Efforts Within The Organization

As earlier managers set about to implement the marketing concept, it became increasingly apparent that it would be impossible to do so "efficiently and effectively" without coordinating efforts across the organization. At first, the focus was simply on coordinating "marketing efforts" within the organization, such as market research, advertising, and sales. This improvement alone was a step forward in the 1950s. However, through the years managers came to understand that it was not just "marketing efforts" that required coordination, but all areas within the organization that have the ultimate goal of fulfilling customer needs. (And, indeed, which areas do not?) These same sentiments toward coordination were echoed in the quality movement admonishments of the 1980s to "break down organizations' functional silos" and to "work and think more cross functionally." In a sense, then, the understanding, creation, and delivery of customer value becomes a unifying vision for the entire organization, the page from which everybody sings.

Achieving Organizations' Ultimate Goals

One of the biggest misperceptions of being customer focused is that it implies a "customer is always right" mentality, where an organization might make decisions that are against its own self-interests. In fact, the marketing concept is very clear that better understanding and serving of customers is *the way* for an organization to achieve its ultimate goals, not a barrier. It suggests that those organizations that best understand customer requirements and that fulfill them more effectively and efficiently than their competitors *will* be the ones who ultimately achieve market success (i.e., longevity, profitability, market share, shareholder value, etc.). The marketing concept aspires to marry the interests of the customer and the organization in a win–win scenario. This perspective also suggests that customers may not always get everything they want or need. Responding to the customer must occur within reason, considering the ultimate welfare of the provider organization. Because if the provider organization cannot achieve its long-term goals of sustainability and profit, customers are the ultimate losers.

In sum, the marketing concept lays out the important philosophical base for organizations that are trying to achieve a stronger marketing focus. However, much more is necessary to implement this concept. With that in mind, the following sections will overview what, exactly, managers (and health care providers) need to know in order to *act,* as well as think, like marketers.

WHAT DO PHYSICIAN LEADERS NEED TO KNOW ABOUT MARKETING?

The responsibility of managers, more than anything else, is to make decisions. *Strategic decisions* are those that result in the deployment of resources that directly influence the conduct and performance of an organization. When many think of marketing, they think about strategic decisions, such as how and where to communicate with customer groups, what products and services to provide, and how to make products/services more accessible and available. However, what many fail to understand is that strategic decisions must first be built upon a foundation; that foundation is the thorough analysis of the organization's market and customer base. In other words, strategic marketing decisions are *preceded* by a physician leader's most important activities—gathering and analyzing market data.

Two frameworks, Market Opportunity Analysis (MOA) and Customer Value Determination (CVD), will be discussed below. Together, these delineate a plan for gathering and analyzing market data, which is critical for physician leaders trying to understand and respond to their dynamic markets and customers. The success of the health care organization's ultimate marketing strategies (regarding promotion, product/service offerings, pricing, etc.) will be directly related to the quality of its MOA and CVD efforts.

MOA

The first question that must be addressed for marketing purposes is "which market(s) are we in?" Indeed, it is only after determining exactly what market you are in, as well as understanding the factors that are shaping the conduct, performance, and viability of that market, that the question of customer value becomes relevant. Conducting a MOA, then, is generally the first marketing skill that must be developed.

Figure 5–1 shows a framework for conducting a MOA. In essence, each of the boxes in the figure represents the collection and analysis of various types of market data. Corresponding strategic decisions must be made along the way in answer to the following types of questions:

- What are the relevant environmental trends that are now, and in the future, going to shape the conduct and performance of this particular market? What factors (relating to change in technology, legal/political, cultural, ecological, or other concerns) will influence the viability of the market, as well as the ability of competitors to respond?
- What is our market definition? Exactly what market are we competing in? What specific products, services, customers, and competitors define the domain of our playing field?
- What do the end-user customers in this market value? What are their requirements, now and in the future? What must organizations know

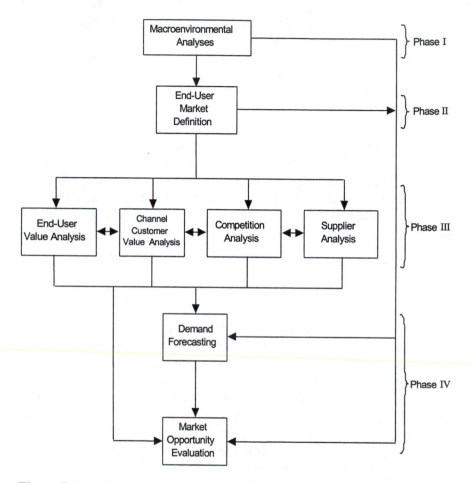

Figure 5–1 Market Opportunity Analysis (MOA) Framework. *Source:* Reprinted with permission from R. Woodruff and S. Gardial, *Know Your Customer: New Approaches to Understanding Customer Value and Satisfaction*, p. 33, © 1996, Blackwell Publishers.

about these customers in order to creatively and effectively be their provider of choice?

- What do we know about other organizations that exist as channel customers? How will their presence alter the way in which we compete in the market?
- How would one evaluate the other competitor/providers in the market? Where are they formidable? Where are they vulnerable?

- What about suppliers in this industry? How do they shape opportunities and constraints for providers?
- What about forecasted demand? How can one quantify current and future opportunities for growth in this market?

In gathering and analyzing the market data that are necessary to answer these questions, marketers begin to understand the parameters of the world in which they wish to compete. In essence, they specify and clarify the playing field, the rules, the constraints, and the opportunities that lie ahead of them. These are tantamount to fleshing out the marketer's "big picture." It is during the analysis of MOA data that one begins to understand what kinds of strategies are more or less likely to be successful for one's organization. MOAs are critical in shaping the direction for future decisions regarding marketing strategies.

CVD

The exploration of customer value is arguably one of the most critical components of any MOA. There are many issues regarding how best to "understand" customers. The CVD process, described below, is the framework that is used in the Physician Executive MBA Program at the University of Tennessee (PEMBA) to guide physician leaders' exploration of their customers' value requirements. Because the pursuit of "customer value" is relatively new to business, a brief history is helpful.

One of the chief tenants of the 1980s quality movement was that organizations should pay more attention to their customers, specifically in the form of aggressively measuring customer satisfaction. Organizations understood that they needed feedback on how they were doing, in order to get an external, customer-driven assessment of their internal quality initiatives. Such customer reports cards were well and good, except managers increasingly found that they fell short of the customer information they needed.

In short, customer satisfaction ratings are a backwards look at what an organization has been doing. Customers are generally asked to evaluate their past experiences and consumption occasions regarding a product and/or service. Unfortunately, many managers desire a forward focus, as well; "What should we do next?" Sole reliance on customer satisfaction measures is, in essence, like trying to drive down a highway by looking in the rear view mirror. Although previously traveled topography, road conditions, and twists and turns might signal what lies ahead, they are a poor substitute for looking out the front window!

As the limitations of customer satisfaction efforts became more apparent, managers in the 1990s increasingly began to focus their attention on customer value (in addition to, not rather than, customer satisfaction). Customer value more accurately captures the notion that organizations need to be constantly looking for new, creative, and superior ways to deliver what customers want and need. In discussing customer value, the following definition has been adopted: Customer value is the customers' perception of what they want to have happen (i.e., consequences) in a specific use situation, with the help of a product or service offering, in order to accomplish a desired purpose or goal (Woodruff & Gardial, 1996).

By taking this definition apart, it becomes more clear what an organization needs to understand about its customers in order to create value for them.

The Customer's Perception

As simplistic as it sounds, managers must accept that customer value is something that must be viewed from the customer's perspective. My experience working with a variety of industries for the past several years has only strengthened my belief that managers do not always see the world in the same way that their customers do. Even more difficult to accept is the notion that customers' perceptions and judgments are often very subjective in nature. Managers will never find a devise to objectively measure whether a product or service is user friendly, comfortable, or makes the customer feel taken care of. Unfortunately, these are precisely the kinds of value dimensions that customers are constantly evaluating about product/service offerings. When we adopt a customer value focus, by definition we move into the customer's world, into their experiences, into their varying use situations and requirements, and into their, often subjective, evaluative criteria.

The Importance of Understanding Consequences

This element of the definition (re)focuses manager's attention on the fact that customers do not simply want products or services, but instead are seeking the *consequences* of having or using them. For example, attractive décor in a doctor's office (attribute) may make the patient feel more relaxed and at ease (consequence). As far as customers are concerned, the specific attributes of products or services are only a means to an end. They are only important in that they allow the customer to experience positive consequences (benefits) that are desired, or that they help him/her avoid or reduce unwanted, negative consequences (costs or sacrifices). In fact, the customer is generally more concerned with *what* s/he experiences than with *how* the provider specifically delivers that experience. The problem with many managers is that they are too attribute focused (on what they provide) rather than being consequence focused (on what the customer experiences). More difficult, still, is the fact that customers' desired consequences are not always explicitly articulated, and the provider must often be aggressive in pursuing and uncovering them.

For example, an emergency department (ED) physician recently related his frustration with patients' family members who continually requested that they interact with only one doctor while their loved ones were in the ED. What these family members articulated (one doctor) was an attribute—something they wanted the provider (hospital) to do and something the physician said the ED was unable to provide. However, this doctor was encouraged to explore the potential consequences underlying the attribute request— *why* did these individuals want to see only one doctor? What was the *consequence* they wanted to experience for which they felt that "one doctor" was the means? Most likely, these family members wished to experience a feeling of confidence regarding the care of their loved ones, an assurance that everything was being handled conscientiously and a belief that nothing was falling between the cracks as multiple care givers came and went from the scene. Understanding that these consequences probably better represent what is really important to family members, the ED staff might then begin to consider what kinds of things (attributes) could be done to create/deliver them. Whereas "one doctor" may not be possible, there may be multiple other responses that could help create the desired consequences: in terms of staffing (e.g., the assignment of a specific, coordinated team of caregivers), processes (e.g., advising family members on how often and to what extent the multiple doctors are communicating with each other), or even symbols (e.g., prominently posting the hospital's quality standards and mission statements). When seen from this perspective, it is truly a focus on customers' consequences that is the key to unlocking customer understanding and, in turn, creating value.

Value is Specific To Use Situations

An important notion in the definition of customer value is that it is situationally driven. In other words, what the customer requires, even of the same product/service provider, can and will vary depending on the particular consumption occasion or situation. For example, a patient's requirements of his/her family physician may be very different on a "well baby" visit than when the child is in distress and seriously ill. In fact, to understand our customers' requirements, we must begin to explore the variety of situations in which customers interact with our products/services, to recognize the value requirements that are unique to those situations, and to formulate potentially different responses to our customers in those situations.

Customers' Desired Purpose or Goals

Finally, the definition recognizes that, aside from the immediate consequences of product/service consumption, all individuals are driven by even higher order desired end states in their lives. Core motivations, or purposes, such as peace of mind, safety and security, being loved by others, and quality of life, are the ultimate ends for which customers strive. These deep-seated and fundamental goals are sometimes even more difficult for customers to articulate than consequences. Nonetheless, we may be sure that product consumption and the resulting consequences are, themselves, only means to these ultimate ends. In fact, the means–end chain that is suggested by the preceding discussion (attributes→consequences→desired end states) has been referred to as "the value hierarchy" and is shown in Figure 5–2.

Seen in this way, it becomes very clear what, exactly, providers need to understand about their customers to create and deliver value. Keeping in mind that different use situations (as well as different customer segments) result in differing value hierarchies, managers can use this framework as the basis for exploring their customers' value requirements. It is interesting to note that while most managers clearly understand the attributes associated with their product or service, they often have less confidence in their understanding of the more important consequences and desired end states, which are motivating their customers, and how these might change in various situations.

It is not within the scope of this chapter to explain exactly how managers should go about generating this type of customer data. Suffice it to say (1) that traditional customer satisfaction measures are rarely adequate in this regard, (2) that the techniques that lead to greater customer value understanding are not rocket science and can be used by virtually any organization, and (3) that it is in the best interests of all managers to make

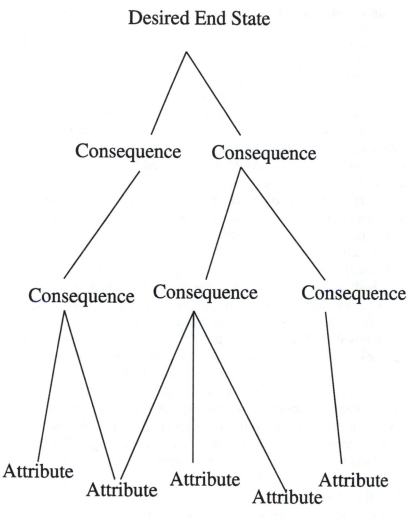

Figure 5–2 Model of a Customer Value Hierarchy

sure their organizations are investing the time and effort it takes to fully explore their customers' value hierarchies. (In fact, in the PEMBA program we have physicians conducting customer value interviews based on only a couple of hours of instruction.) Physician leaders who do not have basic customer value knowledge will find it difficult to move forward and make the subsequent strategic marketing decisions that are required of their organization.

Customer Value As a Unifying, Cross-Functional Orientation

Armed with the knowledge generated from MOA, including a thorough determination of customer value, the physician leader will proceed to make a series of decisions that determine how, exactly, his/her organization will compete within the marketplace. These decisions, and understanding how to make them, typically make up the bulk of marketing texts. Table 5–1 is an overview of the critical strategic decisions that marketers must make. These are listed in their logical ordering, as some decisions should necessarily precede others. In addition, an attempt has been made to highlight specific marketing knowledge/skills that are needed for each decision, as well as an indication of other managers within the organization with whom these decisions should be coordinated. Several points must be made regarding this table.

First, Table 5–1 is rather daunting, considering the number of decisions, their complexity, and the knowledge required to make them. There are many bodies of knowledge that have been developed to help managers deal with the variety of marketing-related strategic decisions that a firm must make. Does a marketing manager need to be expert in all of them? Is it even possible? The answer to both of these questions is, probably not. The marketing manager may have or acquire some of the needed knowledge, may buy this expertise by employing individuals with specific skills, or may outsource some of these decisions to third-party consultants or other organizations (e.g., market research firms, advertising agencies).

What, then, must a good marketer know to coordinate and oversee all of these efforts? As Table 5–1 shows, at a minimum a good marketer must understand the "big picture," which is represented in the MOA and CVD process. The data and analyses from these frameworks provide the foundation for all subsequent marketing decisions. Then, the marketer should have the managerial skills to coordinate the various efforts, in and out of the organization, which must combine to create an integrated, strategically synergistic response to the marketplace. Certainly, a minimal level of understanding regarding each of the marketing decisions in Table 5–1 is important. But marketing managers must also know when to call in experts in the different areas.

The second point that is apparent from the table is the extent to which marketers must interact with various other areas and managers in the organization to put strategies into motion. The efficient and effective coordination that was discussed earlier relative to the marketing concept is a

Table 5–1 Strategic Marketing Decisions

Decision Type	Results In . . .	Specific Marketing Skills Needed	Other Managers/Areas Involved
Setting Market-Level Objectives	Decisions regarding major organizational goals and objectives relative to the market, e.g., level of market penetration, market share objectives, etc.	MOA and CVD analyses	Sr. level managers
Selecting Target Markets	Prioritization of customer segments, resulting in strategic focus on one or a small number of the segments	MOA and CVD analyses, strengths and weaknesses analysis of the provider organziation, targeting strategies	Sr. level managers and unit heads
Segmentation Strategies	Strategic decisions regarding the appropriate marketing mix responses and resources allocated to one or more segments	MOA and CVD analyses, segmentation strategy frameworks, and theory	Marketing research, Sr. level managers and unit heads
Positioning Strategies	Statement of how the provider organization should be perceived by	MOA and CVD analyses, positioning strategy theory, buyer behavior theory	Marketing Research, Sr. level managers and unit heads, Advertising and PR

continues

107

Table 5–1 continued

Decision Type	Results In . . .	Specific Marketing Skills Needed	Other Managers/Areas Involved
	customers relative to the market competitors, in terms of defining characteristic(s) and/or differential marketplace advantage.		
Determining Product/Service Offering	Strategic decisions regarding the combination of products/services to provide, how to provide them, implementation strategies, and elimination processes	MOA and CVD analyses, services marketing theory, Product Life Cycle strategies, New Product Development proceses	Sr. level managers, unit heads, department heads
Promotions Strategy	An integrated strategy involving all elements of the organization's communications with constituencies	MOA and CVD analyses, Advertising, PR, sales, promotions theory and strategies	Advertising, PR, corporate communications, sales
Distribution Strategy	Decisions regarding access to and availability of product/services, including site locations, types of services available, hours of operation, etc.	MOA and CVD analyses, Distribution strategies	Sr. level managers, unit heads, corporate strategic planning

Pricing Strategy	Decisions regarding the pricing structure for products and services	MOA and CVD analyses, Pricing strategy	Sr. level managers, Unit heads, CFO
Post-MOA Alterations in Customer Feedback and Monitoring	Improvements or changes in MOA/CVD efforts to continuously monitor customer perceptions and decision processes and to disseminate that knowledge throughout the organization	MOA and CVD analyses, market research, customer value theory, customer satisfaction theory	Market research, patient services, "complaint" processes
Customer Responsiveness Training For Staff	Efforts to train all relevant staff on customer responsive philosophy, customer value, and corporate objectives and strategies regarding customers, also performance evaluations and reward criteria relevant to customer focus	MOA and CVD analyses, customer value theory, customer satisfaction, the Marketing Concept	Sr. level management, human resources

critical reality. The other managers identified in Table 5–1 represent only general suggestions. Within any specific organization, job titles may vary, and additional or different managers might be required to achieve the cross-functional coordination that is required to implement various marketing strategies. However, Table 5–1 provides a starting point to think about the amount and type of coordination that is needed.

Third, it should be clear from Table 5–1 that all of the marketing strategies are unified by a common vision—that supplied by the MOA and the CVD analysis. While various, seemingly independent, decisions are being made by marketing managers all of the time, in fact, these decisions should all be moving in the same direction. They should all be moving toward the common vision of who the customer is and what the customer requires. If all decisions regarding new services, advertising, customer responsiveness training, pricing, and the like are based upon a common vision of customers' value requirements, then they cannot help but to be synergistic.

Finally, this author's opinion is that most marketing texts, and many programs, have it backwards in terms of emphasis. Most spend a disproportionate amount of time and space on the issues included in Table 5–1, and not nearly enough time on the two analyses that should precede them, namely MOA and CVD. If these two analyses have been covered well in an executive MBA program, then many of the subsequent marketing strategy decisions in Table 5–1 will be more apparent. Likewise, if marketing decisions represent a real struggle for managers; it may be precisely because they do not understand the basics of their market(s) and their customers before they begin. In short, more time spent on the front end marketing analyses greatly facilitates effort on the back end strategic decisions. This point holds, as well, for the desirable content in an executive MBA program for physicians.

THE IMPORTANCE OF MOA AND CVD FOR PHYSICIAN LEADERS

Hopefully, this chapter has provided a compelling discussion about why physician leaders need to understand marketing, as well as what they should know about it. It seems clear that many organizations are eagerly searching for ways to carve out a niche in the ever-changing health care industry, to break down traditional thinking, which revolves around organizational silos or smokestacks, and to identify avenues for real, sustainable competitive advantage in the marketplace. The marketing concept, along with MOA and CVD, provides important responses to these concerns. If health care organizations are to be truly customer focused (and not just pay lip service to it), then it is clear that marketing will require a critical place in the physician leaders' repertoire. While health care organizations will, no doubt, continue to struggle with how to bring the marketing perspective more fully into their organizations, it is certain that they will benefit from the wealth of knowledge the marketing discipline embodies. No doubt, the marketing discipline will also grow and benefit, as it seeks to address the complex challenges of this dynamic service industry.

GLOSSARY

consumers. the end users who actually consume or use the product/service. In health care, the patient is generally considered the ultimate consumer.

customers. organizations or individuals downstream in the value chain through which the provider must sell its services to reach its end users. Health care examples would include insurance companies and patients' employers, both of whom buy but do not ultimately consume, the physician's services.

customer value. customer value is the customers' perception of what they want to have happen (i.e., consequences) in a specific use situation, with the help of a product or service offering, in order to accomplish a desired purpose or goal.

marketing concept. the marketing concept holds that the key to achieving organizational goals consists of determining the needs and wants of target markets and delivering the desired satisfactions more effectively and efficiently than competitors. There are three key elements underlying this definition: (1) the need to understand customers, (2) the need to coordinate efforts within an organization, and (3) the achievement of an organization's ultimate goals, including profitability, ROI, shareholder value, and so on.

marketing mix. traditional marketing texts refer to these four types of decisions which are central to carrying out an organization's strategic marketing plan, including decisions regarding (1) the product/service offering, (2) promotional strategies, (3) distribution, and (4) pricing.

market opportunity analysis. a framework to help marketers logically and systematically understand the factors that are shaping the conduct, performance, and viability of their chosen market(s), including macro environmental trends, target market identification, competitor analysis, customer value determination, supplier analysis, and demand forecasting.

REFERENCES

California group publishes ranking of physicians based on patient surveys. (1997, September 17). *Wall Street Journal*, B6.

Cooper, P. (1994). *Health care marketing*. Gaithersburg, MD: Aspen Publishers.

Drucker, P. (1973). *Management: Tasks, responsibilities, practice.* New York: Harper & Row.

Hansen, H. (1977). *Marketing text and cases*. Homewood, IL: Irwin Publishing Co.

Herzlinger, R. (1997). *Market driven health care.* Reading, MA: Addison-Wesley Publishing Co.

Hosansky, T. (1997, September/October) Opening doctors' ears: How to make CME work in an outcomes-driven world. *Medical Meetings, 24*, 32–39.

How good is your HMO? (1997, November 10). *Business Week*, 107.

Isaacs, S.L., & Schwartz, A.C. (1992) . *The consumer's legal guide to today's health care: Your medical rights and how to assert them.* New York: Houghton Mifflin.

Kotler, P. (1994). *Marketing management: Analysis, planning, implementation and control* (8th ed.). Engelwood Cliffs, NJ: Prentice Hall.

Levitt, T. (1960). Marketing myopia. *Harvard Business Review, July–August*, 45–56.

Miller, C. (1994) Hospitals boost marketing expenses by 25%. *Marketing News, 30*(13), 2.

National health expenditures as a percent of GDP. (1997). Health Care Financing Administration, Office of the Actuary, National Health Statistics Group. Reprinted from *Health Care Financing Review, 19*, 1.

See the doctor, get a toaster. (1997, Dec. 8). *Business Week,* p. 86.

Tracking health care costs: An update. (1997, July/August). *Health Affairs*, 151–155.

Woodruff, R.B., & Gardial, S.F. (1996). *Know your customer: New approaches to understanding customer value and satisfaction.* Boston, MA: Blackwell Business Publications.

PART II

Business Processes and Systems for Financial Stability

CHAPTER 6

Measuring Business Performance

Bruce K. Behn

TABLE OF CONTENTS

EXECUTIVE SUMMARY

What do physician leaders really need to understand about accounting, financial statements, and costing to ask the right questions? How can physician leaders use this information to strategically run their business? How do these concepts integrate with other business disciplines such as marketing, operations, and strategy? These are the questions that will be addressed in this chapter and should be a critical component of any Executive MBA program. Remember, what gets measured gets managed!

FINANCIAL STATEMENTS

Why Do Physician Leaders Need an Understanding of Accounting?

"There were some early hints that all wasn't well at Oxford (Oxford Health Plans, Inc.), despite its robust earnings reports and bullish statements. Early in 1997, for example, it handed in a curious report to New York regulators: a balance sheet that did not balance. The paperwork said the net worth of Oxford's New York HMO subsidiary was $137.2 million, but the numbers added up to less than half that. Over several months, more than $70 million in premiums owed to Oxford had been booked and counted twice. October 27, 1997, Oxford discloses third quarter loss of up to $69.3 million and its stock plunges 62%." (Winslow & Paltow, 1998)

Could you have detected this problem earlier based on your knowledge of financial information? For most non-financial managers, any time accounting and financial statements are mentioned they usually break out in a cold sweat and head toward the aspirin bottle. Why do accounting and financial statements instill the fear of a *60 Minutes* crew arriving at your door? This author's guess is that not only are the statements incomprehensible (written in a foreign language) but also when individuals ask for help deciphering the statements people usually end up more confused than they started. Well accounting is not really a miracle, even though many people think it is!

Accounting is the basic language of business. Every paradigm has its own particular language and set of rules, especially the medical field, and to play in that arena you need to understand both. The only way to accomplish this feat is to have a basic comprehension of the language. Do physician leaders need to understand concepts such as debits or credits? No, but they do need to understand how financial statements are created and how the income statement, balance sheet, and statement of cash flows articulate with one another. They also need to understand some of the underlying assumptions that are used to develop the financial statements.

Accounting is not an exact science. While financial statements are produced under the authoritative guidelines of generally accepted accounting procedures (GAAP), there are some issues you should understand about financial statements. A majority of the numbers in the financial statements are based on estimates. Yes, that is right. Probably the only really hard number on the financial statements is cash. All the others are based on some sort of management estimates. It is like a group of people looking at Sears Tower and asking how tall is this building? How many different guesses would you receive? On average, the group would probably be pretty close but not exact. To become more precise the group would have to exert more time and energy. The same is true of financial statements. There is always a trade-off between more accurate information and the cost to produce this information.

Another assumption GAAP is based on is materiality. Have you ever looked at a set of published financial statements to determine how the numbers are presented? The numbers are usually rounded to the nearest million or billion? Why is this? Once, long ago, this author worked as an auditor for a large accounting firm. On the first job, this auditor found an error that was made to the income statement for approximately 1.3 million dollars. This rookie auditor thought he was in auditor heaven. He went to his senior and joyously explained his findings. Much to his dismay, he was told not to bother the senior again for such insignificant amounts. This rookie auditor was amazed that a 1.3 million dollar error was of no concern to this individual. As the senior explained, this error was just not material to the organization as a whole. So not only are the numbers presented in financial statements rounded to the nearest million/billion, but also the statements audited by accounting firms are only materially correct. That is why if you ever examine an audit opinion the auditors usually say something like the following: In our opinion, the financial statements referred to above present fairly, in all material respects, the consolidated financial position of company and subsidiaries at December 31, 1998 and 1997, and the consolidated results of their operations and their cash flows for each of the three years in the period ended December 31, 1998, in conformity with generally accepted accounting principles.

GAAP is also by nature conservative. Companies can not include the value of customer lists on their balance sheets. Firms also can not show, for the most part, the appreciated market value of its assets. Why is this? Well, how much value would you place on your customer lists? Would an independent third party ascertain the identical value you placed on the asset? Thus, intangible assets such as customer lists do not appear on financial statements unless someone (or a company) buys the assets in an actual transaction. The same is true for appreciating assets. Since market values are difficult to determine, accountants usually use historical cost transactions to develop the financial statements.

While there are many other accounting assumptions that influence the way financial statements are developed, it is important that physician leaders understand that while accounting financial statements provide valuable information, they need to be aware of the assumptions that were used to prepare them. Accounting still provides valuable data that is reliable, comparable, and consistent.

What Is It Physician Leaders Really Need To Understand About Financial Statements?

A CEO of a major corporation once referred to looking at the company's annual financial statements as reading a history book. By the time the annual financial statements are produced, the information provided is useless. This statement may be exaggerating the case somewhat but the point is on target. What if you were told to bowl one game each day for 90 days and then you were to receive a report 45 days later that gave you a total score for your 90 days. However, there is one restriction on the games you bowl. A blanket must be placed in front of the pins; therefore, you are unable to determine how many pins you knocked down each time. Then you were asked to improve your score—could you? (Kaplan & Norton, 1998) This author thinks physician leaders may find this somewhat difficult to do.

Just as you would find it difficult to improve your bowling score, if you receive financial information in an aggregated untimely fashion, it is probably going to be difficult to improve your company's financial performance. Therefore, financial data must be timely to provide us with the ability to assess future cash flows and assist in decision making (an information role) and to monitor debt covenants and bonus arrangements (a stewardship role).

The basic financial statements include the balance sheet, income statement, and statement of cash flows. The balance sheet measures the financial condition of a company at a given point in time, for example December 31, 1998. The income statement and statement of cash flows measure company results for a given period of time, for example for the year ended December 31, 1998.

How do you get a handle on how financial statements articulate with one another without taking five years of accounting and learning all the new vernacular such as debits and credits? The approach the author uses is through simple mathematical equations. Most everyone can understand the basic mathematical laws of addition and subtraction. If you can handle this, you can understand the miracle of accounting. Let us start by looking at the balance sheet as an equation at the end of a period:

$$\text{Assets} = \text{Liabilities} + \text{Owners' Equity.}$$

Most of us can grasp what an asset is, something the company owns that has a monetary value such as cash, equipment, and buildings. What this equation says is that all company assets accumulated throughout the years are owned (or claimed) by someone. A portion of the assets are claimed by creditors (e.g., liabilities) and some of the assets are claimed by the owners (e.g., owners' equity). So if assets equal $100,000, liabilities equal $30,000, and owners' equity equals $70,000 then this equation should be in balance. Is it, $100,000 = $30,000 + $70,000? Yes, looks good so far! But does this equality always hold?

If we expand the owners' equity portion of this equation, we can now include the summary result of the income statement (net income)

$$\text{Owners' Equity (Ending)} = \text{Owners' Equity (Beginning)}$$
$$+ \text{ Net Income} - \text{Dividends}$$

and since Net Income equals Revenues minus Expenses we now have an equation that can demonstrate how the financial statements are linked together:

$$\text{Assets} = \text{Liabilities} + \text{Owners' Equity (Beginning)}$$
$$+ \text{ Revenues} - \text{Expenses} - \text{Dividends.}$$

If beginning owners' equity is $60,000, revenues are $300,000, expenses are $270,000, and dividends $20,000, does this equality balance?

$$\$100,000 = \$30,000 + \$60,000 + \$300,000 - \$270,000 - \$20,000.$$

Yes it does.

Why Is It Important That We Understand How The Different Financial Statements Work Together?

In most businesses, there is at least one accounting performance measure that is used to evaluate its performance and it usually has something to do with net income (or earnings). If you look at Figure 6–1, most companies still use earnings based numbers for performance measurement and compensation. For example, return on assets (ROA) and return on owners' equity (ROE) are common ratios that are used to assess a company's progress, as the basis for incentive pay, and to benchmark progress against other firms. Return in these ratios is measured by net income. Given the accounting equation example above, ROA would be ($300,000 − $270,000) / $100,000 or 30%. ROE would be $30,000/$70,000 or approximately 43%.

Let us use these ratios to understand how the decisions we make flow through the accounting financial statements and ultimately influence the ratio ROA. What if you had a decision to buy, on credit, new equipment that costs $4000 but that would save $2,000 per year in costs? How would the accounting equation and, ultimately, the financial ratios be effected? Well, assets must increase by $4000 and liabilities must also go up $4000 because we still owe this money as a liability, so the accounting equation would look like this (notice everything is still in balance):

$$\$104,000 = \$34,000 + \$60,000 + \$300,000 - \$270,000 - \$20,000.$$

But we also saved some money because our expenses decreased by $2,000 and therefore cash also increased by $2,000. Does the equation still balance? Let's see,

$$\$106,000 = \$34,000 + \$60,000 + \$300,000 - \$268,000 - \$20,000.$$

Guess what? The accounting equation still holds. See, it is truly a miracle.

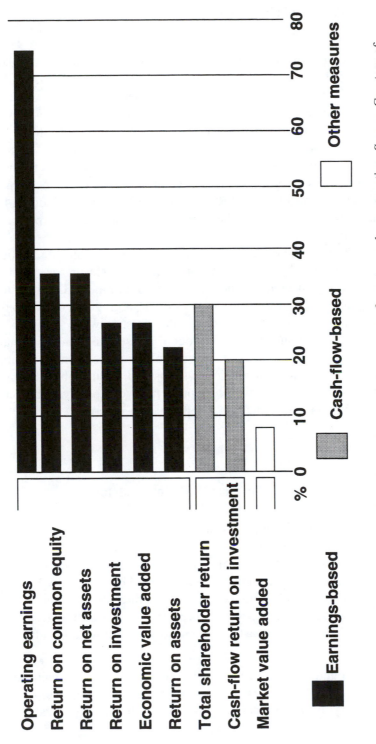

Figure 6–1 Percent of companies using these financial measures to assess performance and compensation. *Source:* Courtesy of Financial Executives Research Foundation, Morristown, New Jersey.

This is a simple example but hopefully you see that this relationship will always hold no matter what transaction you are trying to analyze. Remember, the important issue here is that you understand enough about accounting and the financial statements that you can ask the right questions. You do not need to understand the intricacies of the accounting–leave that up to your accountant. As a final step, let us determine how our changes would influence our ROA and ROE ratios. If we now look at the financial ratios given the changes we made, what happened? ROA is now $32,000/$106,000 or 30.2% and ROE is now $32,000/$72,000 or 44.4%. See what happened? At least in the short term this appears to have been a good decision.

Now we have a basic understanding of how financial statements articulate with one another and how to measure financial performance. We need to take this a step further and look at the costs within the organization. Most companies have a fairly good handle on aggregate costs because they are summarized for the financial statements. However, if you start disaggregating costs and start asking detail questions about how much this service or contract costs you usually get blank stares. Getting accurate cost data from company information systems is difficult at best for most companies. Therefore, as the world becomes more competitive it becomes more important that companies get a better handle on costs.

COSTING

Why Is Getting A Handle On Costs Still So Important?

> "Big employers, fuming over demands for steep rate increases for health coverage, are stepping up pressure on health maintenance organizations and healthcare providers to cut costs the way the rest of American industry has done. You have to look at the cost side, says Ken Francese, executive director for compensation and benefits at Chrysler Corp. People in health care say there is 20% to 30% waste in the system." (White & Rundle, 1998)

Does this sound familiar? Health care costs are going up again. Some experts predict that health care costs are expected to increase 4-5% in 1998. So everyone is now hammering on health care organizations to

Table 6–1 Why Focus on Costs?

Firm	A	B	5% revenue incr. A	5% revenue incr. B	5% cost decr. A	5% cost decr. B
Revenues	100	100	105	105	100	100
Costs	– 80	– 90	– 84	– 94.5	76	85.5
Profits	20	10	21	10.5	24	14.5
			5%	5%	20%	45%

lower costs again. Why does corporate management appear to always concentrate on reducing costs rather t han finding ways to bring in more revenue? Table 6–1 shows that if costs are greater than 50% of revenues you get a greater return from decreasing costs than from increasing revenues. When costs are less than 50% of revenues, then increasing revenues will produce a more favorable effect than reducing costs. Guess what the current situation is in the health care industry?

Not only is reducing overall costs important but also improving the accuracy of costing information is becoming more critical to enhancing company performance. Indirect costs are becoming a larger portion of company overall costs. As indirect costs become a larger portion of overall costs it becomes more important that these costs are allocated accurately. In most cases, the information received from company costing systems is of very little value to you in making strategic decisions for the organization. Yes, you have information to satisfy auditors and receive your reimbursements (and sometimes this doesn't even work very well), but you do not have the requisite information to accurately accumulate what a particular managed care contract or particular procedure is costing you?

Traditional costing procedures would allocate these indirect costs based on some sort of volume measure. When this occurs, the highest volume (usually lowest complexity) departments or procedures get hit with the largest percentage of costs, even though this department or procedure may not actually be using (or absorbing) that amount of indirect costs. Therefore, a cross-subsidy of costs occurs, where one department or procedure although very complex by nature (but low volume) absorbs very little indirect costs. These cross-subsidies of service costs can cause all sorts of disrupting behavior in organizations.

How Can We Develop More Accurate Costs?

Do you have a set of financial statements that look like Exhibit 6–1?

What does this tell you about the way your business is operating—not much? What other types of information would you like to know? Would the income statement in Exhibit 6–2 be more informative to you?

Activity based costing can provide you with the necessary information you need to address the critical questions you need to run your business. Activity Based Costing (ABC) is based on a very simple yet very powerful principle: activities consume resources and products or services consume the output of these activities. ABC focuses on the management and cost of activities whereas traditional costing systems focus on departmental and product or service costs. ABC improves the costing of products/services by more accurately assigning overhead or indirect costs on a cause-and-effect basis. Even with all the current hospital consolidation, industry experts still estimate that 20 to 25% of all hospitals are still losing money and need creative ways to keep out of the red. Activity based costing can help in this endeavor.

As Judith Baker points out, "There is a need for ABC in health care because competition is driving down costs while productivity and efficiency remain serious concerns. ABC can deliver the information to maximize

---

Exhibit 6–1 Financial Statement

Health System Inc.
Income Statement
For the period ending December 31, 1998

Revenues:	1200
Operating Expenses:	
Salaries	550
Benefits	100
Supplies	100
Other	50
Total Operating Expenses	800
Contribution Margin	400
Depreciation	100
Excess of Revenue over Expense	300
(or Net Income or earnings)	
Percent Return on Revenues	25%

Exhibit 6–2 Income Statement

Health System Inc.
Income Statement
For the period ending December 31, 1998

	Client #1	Client #2	Total
Revenues:			
Claims Administration	400	300	700
Formulary Rebate	200	100	300
Capitation	100	100	200
Total Revenue	700	500	1200
Expenses:			
Obtain Clients	30	10	40
Implement New Clients	5	0	5
Manage Plans	25	20	45
Produce Cards	10	30	40
Maintain Eligibility	45	30	75
Process Claims	50	120	170
Manage Clients	10	20	30
Manage Client Products	35	10	45
Manage Clinical Programs	10	0	10
Produce Reports	20	30	50
Process Internal Documents	20	20	40
Support Clients	20	0	20
Manage Pharmacy Networks	50	0	50
Develop and Improve Processes	10	5	15
Develop Products and Programs	30	40	70
Understand Markets and Customers	20	20	40
Support Human Resources	30	15	45
Financial Administration	20	70	90
Facilities Administration	10	10	20
Total Expenses	450	450	90
Net Income by Client	250	50	300
Percent Return on Revenues	36%	10%	25%

resources and to relate costs to performance and outcomes measures. Management can use ABC information to accomplish cost efficiency without negatively impacting the quality of service delivery." (Baker, 1998)

How does activity based costing work? As outlined in Figure 6–2, resources are first allocated to activities and these activity costs are allo-

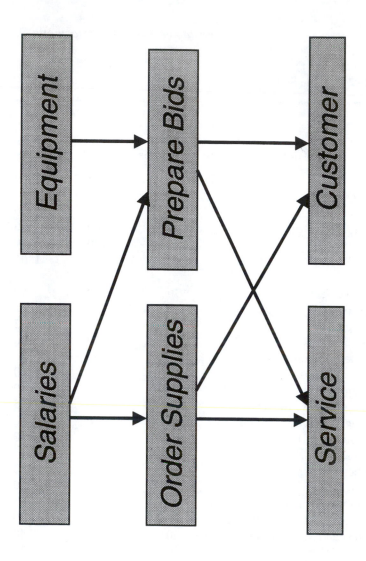

Resources:
How much do we spend?

Activities:
What we do?

Cost objects:
For whom or for what do we do work?

Figure 6–2 Activity Based Costing Vocabulary

126

cated to cost objects such as service or customer costs. This appears simple enough—let's try an example. Exhibits 6–3 and 6–4 outline a simple example using a pharmacy. Notice if we would just look at the typical financial statements, all you would see is $1000 for salary expense. Using ABC we now can see what the pharmacy actually does rather than just what is spent on salaries: take orders ($200 = 20% × $1,000), do administration ($300 = 30% × $1,000), and prepare doses ($500 = 50% × $1,000). Now we can allocate these activities to our cost objects pills and special mixtures. Notice the differences in cost in the two products under traditional costing versus ABC costing. Under traditional costing, both products costs $2.85 per dose. Under ABC, the pills cost $1.30 and the special mixtures cost $12.20 per dose, because the special mixtures are more complex to make and take more time. Although this is a simple example, this author thinks it gives you a feeling of the potential that ABC costing has to provide critical information you need to run your business.

BUSINESS INTEGRATION

How Can We Possibly Keep Track Of Everything That Is Going On In Our Organizations?

Can one financial metric really depict what is going on in my organization? Can a ratio such as return on equity really evaluate whether the

---

Exhibit 6–3 ABC Example: Pharmacy Department

Salary Costs From General Ledger		$1000
What do the pharmacists do:		
Take Orders	20%	
Do Administration	30%	
Prepare Doses	50%	

	Pills	Special Mixtures
Number of Orders	90	10
Time Spent on Paperwork	20%	80%
Time Spent on Preparation	30%	70%
Number of Doses	300	50

What would appear in the financial statements for pharmacy?

Exhibit 6–4 ABC Example: Pharmacy Department

Using ABC methodology what would the pharmacy activity report look like?

		Pills	Special Mixtures
Take Orders	$200	180	20
Do Administration	$300	60	240
Prepare Doses	$500	150	350
	$1,000	$390	$610
Number of Doses		300	50
Cost Per Dose—ABC		$1.30	$12.20
Cost Per Dose—Traditional		$2.85	$2.85

strategic initiatives undertaken in my organization are really working? This author does not think so. For one thing, ratios based on accounting financial statements are founded on historical information that tell you very little about the future direction of the company. In addition, does a simple ratio really summarize how well the fundamental value drivers of your organization are working? Using the analogy of a ship, how would you like to be steering the *Titanic* with only information on the speed of the ship and without having any information on wind conditions, fuel, direction, or other weather conditions such as icebergs. You would never do this, so why would you look at your organization in that way. What you would like to have is real-time information on where you have been and where you are going on a number of dimensions. That is why Kaplan and Norton some years ago suggested that management should start using a balanced approach to running their firms (Kaplan & Norton, 1996).

While some companies have developed market based measures (such as economic value created) to evaluate and strategically run their organizations, this author finds these are conceptually pleasing but difficult to roll out throughout the organization. How does an admitting clerk understand that improving what he/she does can actually impact an overall measure such as economic value created? The *Balanced Scorecard* approach initiated by Kaplan and Norton provides a common sense way to perform this task.

How would you, as the physician leader, translate the following vision/mission statement into operationalized objectives that can be cascaded down throughout the entire organization. In our pursuit of our vision, we have grown, changed, adapted, and reinvented ourselves—to meet the challenges of our competition, to take advantage of innovation, and to deliver on the dreams and demands of our customers. We continue to be committed to outstanding products, solid operations, and long-term shareholder value. Sounds good but how do you translate this into an action plan that employees can understand? The *Balanced Scorecard* provides executives with a comprehensive framework that translates a company's vision and strategy into a coherent set of performance metrics.

As Kaplan and Norton point out, the *Balanced Scorecard* emphasizes that financial and nonfinancial measures must be part of the information system for all levels of the organization. All employees must understand the financial consequences of their decisions and actions; senior executives must understand the drivers of long-term financial success. The metrics for the *Balanced Scorecard* are more than just a collection of financial and nonfinancial performance measures; they are driven by the mission and strategy. The *Balance Scorecard* should translate a company's mission and strategy into tangible objectives and measures. The measures should represent a balance between external measures and internal measures and between the results from past experience and the measures that drive future performance. Finally, the scorecard should be balanced between objective, quantifiable outcome measures and subjective, judgemental performance drivers of outcome measures (Kaplan & Norton, 1996).

How Do We Begin To Understand How To Integrate All This Business Knowledge?

How do you obtain experience integrating these business concepts without having to first experiment on an actual company? We have found that the best way to accomplish this feat is through interactive simulations. If simulations can mimic the real world business environment including all the uncertainty and complex business decisions, they can provide real world experience in the safe environment of a simulation. It appears we have discovered a simulation that meets the test, *The Marketplace*. As one executive who completed the simulation exerted, "*The Marketplace* even for those of us with considerable industry experience, the results of the game seemed real. We believed that the results were driven by our strategies and tactics and that we were the masters of our own destiny. Success or failure, market share and profits, were all driven by our ability to interpret signals from our customers and develop strategies that met those needs. It was the epiphany that took the discipline of strategic marketing from an academic exercise to reality." (Cadotte & Bruce, 1998)

The Physician Executive MBA program culminates with this very intensive business simulation, called *The Marketplace*, which was developed by 10 faculty at the University of Tennessee. Ernie Cadotte (marketing professor at The University of Tennessee) and Harry Bruce (former CEO of the Illinois Central Railroad) joined forces with this multidisciplinary team to create this computerized simulation, called *The Marketplace*.

As Cadotte and Bruce point out

> "*The Marketplace* is a comprehensive business simulation which integrates all functional areas of business. Players start up and run their own company, struggling with business fundamentals and the interplay between marketing, manufacturing, finance, accounting and management. The consequences of the players' decisions are quickly reflected in the simulated marketplace. By studying end user opinions, competitor decisions, and their own financial performance, the players learn to adjust their strategy to become stronger competitors. Over the course of the entire exercise, the players' understanding of the linkages among the functional areas of business grows at an exponential rate." (Cadotte & Bruce, 1998)

In order to manage playing the simulation within the semester, we compress time and speed up the business cycle, then immerse the players in the management of business. In eight decision rounds representing 2 years of compressed time, players evaluate the market opportunity, choose a business strategy, evaluate the tactical options and make a series of decisions with profitability in mind. The players' decisions are combined with the decisions of the student teams and run through a simulated marketplace. The results are fed back to the players for the next round of decision making.

Why Use A Simulation?

According to Cadotte and Bruce there are five hallmarks to the simulation methodology that really make it work: a heavy emphasis on the interconnectedness of the business disciplines; the continuous application of strategic planning and execution skills; persistent focus on bottom line profitability while simultaneously delivering customer value; the repetitive practice of budgeting and cash-flow management; and a strong emphasis on leadership, teamwork and interpersonal skills.

The learning strategy is to gradually build the business and thus, gradually introduce new issues that must be mastered by the players. Each quarter or decision period has a dominant activity and a set of decisions that are linked to it. These dominant activities take the players through the business life cycle from start-up, to development, to growth, and ultimately to near maturity. Each quarter's activities not only result in new material being introduced, but also build upon the prior content so that there is considerable repetition. Business activities such as cash flow planning, value creation in product design, scheduling, profitability analysis, and strategic planning and management require repetitive exercise in order to set them into the natural thinking of the players.

Another major strength of the simulation is its emphasis on strategic planning and execution. The chief advantage of the simulation is that the player must continually develop a strategy for the current period while always positioning the firm for the future (the longer-term strategy). Moreover, the situation is constantly changing so that each decision period represents a new situation to be analyzed and a need to skillfully adjust the strategy for the future.

The players begin by analyzing market research data in order to understand their market and customers. Based on this information the participants must design products to reach their target markets. To support these new brands, the players must devise advertising campaigns, sales force incentives, and price options and services. In the first four quarters of the game, every team (management) invests four million dollars of their own money. However, four millions dollars is not enough capital to sustain growth. So all teams must try to obtain venture capital money to continue growing their companies. Before quarter five begins, we simulate a venture capitalists fair by having UT faculty and PhD students pose as venture capitalists. The players must prepare and present a business plan to the venture capitalists. The players try to obtain an additional five million of capital in the open market in exchange for shares of their company. However, there is a shortage of capital and all teams will not receive five million dollars. In addition, teams do not want to lose control of their company. You can imagine what a very exciting and emotional day this is.

As the game continues, players must allocate scarce funds to research and development (R&D), marketing, advertising, and distribution and select and prioritize R&D of new product and service features. Throughout the simulation the players must forecast demand, manage cash, compete heat-to-head with other business teams, thereby honing the teams ability to adjust strategy and tactics in response to financial performance and competitive tactics.

GLOSSARY

accounting. the process that culminates in the preparation of financial or managerial reports for an organization for use by parties both internal or external to the enterprise.

balance sheet. provides information about an organization's investments, obligations, and owners' equity at a given point in time.

financial statements. the principal means through which financial information is communicated to those parties external to the organization.

generally accepted accounting procedures. a common set of accounting standards and procedures adopted by the accounting profession.

income statement. a report that measures revenues and expenses of an organization for a given period of time.

materiality. a qualitative characteristic of accounting information that means an amount, because of its size or importance, would influence the decision of an investor.

return on assets. net income for the year divided by total assets at the end of the same year.

return on owners' equity. net income for the year divided by total owner's equity at the end of the same year.

statement of cash flows. provides information about an organization's cash receipts and cash payments for a given a period of time.

REFERENCES

Baker, J. (1998). *Activity based costing and activity based management.* Gaithersburg, MD: Aspen Publishers.

Cadotte, E., & Bruce, H. (1998). *The management of strategy in the marketplace.* Knoxville, TN: University of Tennessee Press.

Kaplan, R., & Norton, D. (1996). *The balanced scorecard—Translating strategy into action.* Cambridge, MA: Harvard Business School.

Kaplan, R., & Norton, D. (1998). *Cause and effect, using integrated cost systems to drive profitability and performance.* Cambridge, MA: Harvard Business School.

White, J., & Rundle, R. (1998, May 19). Big companies fight health-plan rates. *Wall Street Journal*, p. A1.

Winslow, R., & Paltow, S. (1998, April 29). Oxford health plans grew with scant heed to financial controls. *Wall Street Journal*, p. A1.

CHAPTER 7

Cash Flow, Expansion, and the Access to Capital

Phillip R. Daves

TABLE OF CONTENTS

EXECUTIVE SUMMARY

The organizational forms under which health care is delivered in this country have changed dramatically during the last decade. Health care organizations will face the new millenium having undergone extensive consolidation and financial restructuring. Consolidation, through acquisitions and mergers, has reduced the number of provider organizations, and financial restructuring has been required to provide the ready access to capital to fund these purchases. Increasingly, the remaining not-for-profit organizations will find themselves with larger and larger debt burdens, and formerly not-for-profit organizations that are purchased by for-profit corporations will find themselves having to focus on the new, and potentially alien, concept of profit. The remaining firms, whether for-profit or not-for-profit, must develop an enhanced awareness of how cash is generated and used.

These organizational changes are the result of growth that cannot be financed with internal funds. Corporate America has known for decades that when debt is used to finance growth, firms lose some of the flexibility to weather financial downturns. Even not-for-profit health care organizations must carefully plan to have enough cash on hand to meet scheduled debt payments, otherwise financial distress may damage their viability. When equity is used in a firm's financing mix, for example when a not-for-profit is bought by a corporation, the resulting firm must ensure that the rate of return on the funds used is sufficiently high to compensate the stockholders. This requires careful forecasting of the costs and benefits of projects by specifically projecting their cash flows *before* investment is undertaken. The more rapid the growth within a firm, the more important is forecasting. Because of this, it is critical that an executive MBA program address the topics of the goal of a public corporation, cash flow estimation, and project selection (also known as capital budgeting).

CAPITAL

An important result of the changes in the delivery and administration of health care in the U.S. is that health care providers, whether individual doctors, stand alone clinics, hospitals, for-profit or not-for-profit, have increasingly found themselves in need of new capital. Health care providers' traditional uses of capital for investment in physical plant, working capital, and equipment have been augmented by investment in information systems, the outright purchase of physician practices, and the establishment of large-scale integrated delivery systems. Internal sources of capital are often inadequate for even the conventional working capital and physical plant needs of a growing health care company. Add to these needs the increased capital demands of integration of services, and the result is the extensive use of debt for some companies, and the use of external equity for other companies.

Internal Capital

A company generates internal capital when it receives more than enough revenue to fund the operating costs associated with doing business. Revenue, which is income from patient fees, insurance payments, and capitation payments, in excess of operating expenses can be used for reinvestment in the firm, such as for equipment purchases, investment in working capital, or maintenance or upgrade of facilities. Some low-growth, high-profit firms find that they can fund all of their required investments in this way. For most growing firms, though, internal funds are not sufficient to meet these capital demands, and health care companies have traditionally resorted to debt financing, contributions, or grants to make up the difference between the capital generated internally and the investment required. During the last decade, though, health care companies have increasingly resorted to outside equity as a source of capital.

External Capital

External capital is used by virtually all large or growing firms. Even small sole proprietorships use external capital in the form of personal bank loans and lines of credit. The primary sources of this capital, debt and equity, have quite different effects on the riskiness, control, and goal of the firm. Because of these differences, the choice of the method of financing is an important decision.

Debt

Various forms of debt such as bank loans, bond issues, and lines of credit have long been the capital mainstay of the health care industry. For small to moderate-sized capital needs that are short-term in nature, bank loans are relatively easy to obtain and have relatively small transaction fees. For larger or longer-term capital needs, bond issues are more commonly used. In either case, the salient features of debt as a source of financing are that:

- scheduled, contractual interest and principal payments must be made by the borrower

- interest payments are tax-deductible
- if the borrower does not make the scheduled contractual payments, then the borrower is in default, and the lender typically has some form of legal recourse
- the lender does not participate in the operation of the company, and has no voting rights.

These characteristics are a double-edged sword for the growing company. The advantage of debt is that control of the firm is not sacrificed and residual earnings do not have to be shared with the lenders (also known as debtholders). So if the company is a for-profit concern and becomes wildly profitable through growth and careful management, the owners of the firm will reap all of the profits in excess of those contractual interest and principal debt payments. If the company happens to be a not-for-profit corporation, then the issuance of debt does not change its not-for-profit status or its mission. On the other hand, if the growing company experiences unforeseen financial difficulties, as almost all companies do from time to time, then there may not be enough cash on hand to make contractual payments to the debtholders. This can be a serious problem. Depending on the type of debt contract that is in place, the debtholders have options at hand to address default that range from restructuring of the debt to repossession of collateral to takeover and liquidation of the firm.

A secured loan is one in which the borrower pledges an asset as collateral for the loan. In the event of default, the debtholder can take possession of the asset and sell it to repay the debt. Mortgages, equipment loans, and auto loans are examples of secured loans. The risk to the borrower of a secured loan is that if the collateral pledged for the loan is essential to the operation of the firm, then in the event of default, the debtholders may repossess that which enables the company to continue operating.

An unsecured loan does not have specific collateral associated with it, but instead relies on the firm's operations for repayment. In the event of default by the borrower, the holder of an unsecured loan can be repaid from the proceeds from liquidating the firm, but only after collateral pledged for other loans is sold or transferred to satisfy those loans.

These possible reactions by debtholders to default can be quite disruptive to a firm that is already in temporary financial trouble. However, in many cases the liquidation value of assets, or of an entire firm, is substantially less than its value as a going concern; debtholders would not receive complete repayment even if the firm were liquidated. For this reason debtholders try to avoid liquidation and repossession and instead often agree to restructure the debt of a firm that is in default by postponing interest payments, reducing the interest rate on the loan, or even taking an equity position in exchange for the debt so that the firm may continue to operate.

Equity

Equity is an ownership interest in the firm. Firms that issue equity sell part ownership in the firm in return for investment capital. Investors pay for an equity position in a company in hopes of making a profit by either receiving their pro rata share of the company's dividends or selling the position later for a profit. Common stock is the certificate that conveys this ownership, and common stockholders are the legal owners of any firm with equity as part of the capital structure. Not the board of directors. Not management. Not the customers. The common stockholders are the owners of the firm.

The equity in some firms is closely held by a few individuals and is not readily available to the public. These private corporations may be owned and managed by the same people. The equity in many other firms is widely held and traded on exchanges like the New York Stock Exchange or Nasdaq. These firms are called public corporations and anyone may purchase shares in these companies and become a partial owner. Stockholders exert control over the public corporation by electing the board of directors, which appoints management, who then run the firm for the benefit of the stockholders. Members of the board of directors or management may also be common stockholders, and hence have an ownership position in the firm, but their positions on the board of directors or management per se do not make them owners.

Companies that resort to equity financing by issuing stock to the public become public, for-profit companies, and the stockholders expect the company to be operated for their benefit. In fact, the ultimate goal of the public corporation is to maximize the value of the stockholder's interest in the company—i.e. management should act in such a way as to maximize the value of the stock. The business headlines of the 1980s and 1990s are filled with examples of managers who ignored this fundamental goal and were ousted by angry stockholders.

The public corporate form has serious implications for the types of activities in which the company will choose to engage. For example, it might be a completely appropriate mission for a private, or not-for-profit, or community-owned hospital to focus the majority of its efforts on delivering high quality uncompensated indigent care, provided that it recovers enough on its fee-based care, or through charity solicitations, to cover ongoing costs and remain financially viable. However such a mission would be completely inappropriate for a public corporation. That is not to say that a corporate-owned hospital cannot or will not provide indigent care. It may be required to do so for a variety of reasons. But the public corporation's obligation is to maximize the financial return to its owners and so must focus on that goal rather than on providing free services. If it is crucial that an organization focus on something other than stockholder wealth maximization, such as providing free medical care, then it should not be organized as a public corporation.

For those companies for which public ownership is appropriate, the great advantage of equity financing relative to debt financing is flexibility. There are no required payments associated with equity, which means that if the firm experiences a temporary downturn or cash shortage, it does not face the added pressure of foreclosure or default. Because of this enhanced flexibility, a firm financed with a large portion of equity can afford to make more risky investments than a firm financed mostly with debt. For this reason, firms in high risk, high growth industries tend to be financed with more equity, while firms in low growth, low risk industries tend to be financed with more debt. Historically, health care delivery has not fit the profile of a high risk, high growth industry, and hence the predominance of not-for-profits and professional corporations. However consolidation in the industry and the competitive pressures unleashed by managed care have increased both the growth and risk of the remaining firms. A result of this industry shift is the increasing presence of public corporations.

The major disadvantage of equity financing for a for-profit firm is dilution of ownership. Issuing equity is by definition selling partial ownership of the firm. The new owners are entitled to a proportional vote, and are entitled to a percentage of the profits that are distributed. These additional votes may hamper the existing owners' ability to control the firm, and will certainly reduce the percentage of profits to which they are entitled.

Equity and the Not-For-Profit

Not-for-profit corporations (as opposed to for-profit corporations that don't happen to make a profit) do not have owners and do not have equity and so do not have access to the equity capital market. These companies have traditionally relied on internal cash flows, debt, and government grants or charitable contributions for investment capital. Recently, though, health care not-for-profits have found themselves unable to acquire sufficient capital through these traditional means to compete effectively in a dynamic health care industry. Unable to expand services and make themselves attractive providers, they have been marginalized in large numbers, with increasing closings and failures. One market response to this phenomenon is the wholesale purchase of not-for-profit health care organizations by for-profit corporations. Columbia HCA is an example of one such public corporation that has purchased many formerly private or not-for-profit hospitals. In a real sense a market experiment is underway in the health care industry with the question asked: What are the advantages of a wholly-owned health care delivery system and do these advantages outweigh the costs imposed by a for-profit ownership structure? The experiment is far from complete.

A complete analysis of the multitude of reasons behind the restructuring of not-for-profit organizations into for-profit corporations, and the impact that this restructuring has on the quality and cost of health care delivery is beyond the scope of this chapter. Instead, a select few of the more important motivations and implications will be discussed.

First, the STARK legislation limits the ability of loosely aligned health care organizations to receive payment for referrals for ancillary services. One of the more obvious effects of this restriction is to encourage the establishment of wholly-owned integrated delivery systems so that ancillary services can be provided, and the revenues realized, within a single organization rather than through referral. This requires the wholesale purchase of hospitals and physician practices and, for the most part, only the public corporation has access to the large sums of equity capital necessary to create this wholly-owned integrated health care delivery system.

Second, the ability to control costs and quality is, in theory, enhanced when the entire chain of operations from primary care physician to inpatient hospital services is owned and operated by the same entity. For example, the health care industry as a whole has been completely unable (or unwilling?) to integrate—or even standardize—information systems across multiple organizations. One of Columbia HCA's goals in purchasing hospital systems is to establish compatible information delivery systems across its entire organization, enabling rapid and efficient access of patient, quality, and outcomes information throughout the entire system.

Third, it is more efficient to provide incentive contracts to managers of a for-profit corporation than a not-for-profit corporation. A for-profit corporation can compensate managers for cutting costs and improving quality by paying them a portion of the added profit that they generate or by tying bonuses into stock price performance. Not-for-profits are limited in their ability to distribute residual income and have no objective measure of firm value such as stock price on which to base performance contracts.

Of course one of the implications of corporate ownership of health care companies is that they must be operated for the benefit of the stockholders. If a community-owned hospital is sold to a for-profit corporation, it will certainly be operated for the benefit of the acquiring stockholders—and the specifics of this operation may well be at odds with the community's wishes. Again, using the indigent care example, a community-owned and subsidized hospital might have a history of providing a great deal of indigent care. As has often been the case, suppose the community decides that it is not willing or able to continue to subsidize the hospital and, instead of closing it, sells it to a for-profit corporation. Once owned by a for-profit corporation, the hospital drastically cuts back its indigent care. Is this what the community wants? Probably not. Is this appropriate behavior for the hospital? Probably. What should the community do to provide indigent care? Remember that the community sold the hospital and received a cash payment in return for the hospital. This money could certainly be used to purchase indigent care at fair market prices from the for-profit hospital. In effect, the community gets out of the hospital business, but remains in the indigent care business. If, instead, the community spends the proceeds from selling the hospital on tax cuts, roads, or other improvements, then the community, not the hospital, is making the decision to cut indigent care.

CASH FLOWS

A firm faced with an expansion project basically has three alternatives: fund the project with internal funds; fund the project with debt; or fund the project with outside equity (a not-for-profit firm can seek grants and donations instead of equity). If internal funds are used for expansion, then their availability over time must be predicted and controlled. If debt is used, there must be sufficient cash available to make scheduled interest and principal payments. If equity is used, then the stockholders expect their money to be invested in ways that earn an appropriate rate of return. Even when a not-for-profit uses donated fund capital for expansion, it must still operate in such a way that it remains financially viable if it hopes to accomplish its mission.

Irrespective of the corporate form—public, private, for-profit, or not-for-profit—each of these funding alternatives requires a careful understanding of the cash flows of the firm as a whole, and the cash flows associated with the proposed expansion. Failure to understand cash flow in any of these cases can result in impaired ability to accomplish the firm's mission, financial distress, or even failure.

Operating Cash Flows

For most firms, cash is generated from operations and from various non-operating assets, such as investments in marketable securities. The first step in identifying the cash flows for a firm is to identify the cash flows generated by operations by calculating net operating profit after taxes (NOPAT). NOPAT is defined as earnings before interest and taxes (EBIT) less the taxes on EBIT:

$$NOPAT = EBIT - \text{Taxes on EBIT}$$
$$= EBIT(1 - \text{Tax rate}).$$

NOPAT is a measure of operating performance that is not affected by the level of debt, or by the level of other non-operating assets. It is the after-tax profit generated by the day to day operations of the firm before taking into account any required reinvestment in the firm, and before taking into account any dividends or required payments on debt.

Depreciation is a line item expense on the income statement that reflects how much a company has "used up" its fixed assets during the year. Although it is treated as an expense, it is not really a cash flow since a company does not really write a check for depreciation payments; the firm just deducts it as if it were really an expense for reporting purposes. Expenses like this that appear on the income statement, but don't really require a cash payment, are called non-cash expenses. These items are incorporated into NOPAT, and so NOPAT understates the cash generated by the firm by this amount. Adding back in non-cash expenses, such as depreciation, results in operating cash flow:

$$
\begin{array}{r}
\text{EBIT} \\
-\underline{\text{Taxes on EBIT}} \\
\text{NOPAT} \\
+\underline{\text{Depreciation}} \\
\text{Operating Cash Flow}
\end{array}
$$

Operating cash flow, plus any non-operating income such as interest income, may be thought of as the pool of internal funds available to pay for debt service, dividends, and any new investment required in the firm. See Figure 7–1. If debt service, dividend payments, and new investment in the firm exceed operating cash flow, then the firm must resort to some form of outside financing as discussed above.

Investments

One of the most costly errors that a growing firm can make is to be careless in planning for expansion. Growth in a firm requires investment, and the faster the growth, the larger the investment required. Every year thousands of profitable firms fail or fall into financial distress because their expansion plans are inadequately funded. For the purpose of this dis-

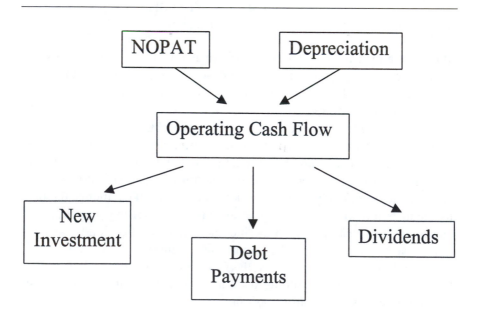

Figure 7–1 Internally Generated Cash Flows

cussion, investments will fall into two categories. The first category is investment in new equipment, buildings, office space and the like. These investments have something physical associated with them and are usually explicitly budgeted for.

The second category is investment in net working capital (NWC). Net working capital is the difference between the short-term assets and short-term liabilities of the firm. For example, a firm might have assets and liabilities on its balance sheet for 1998 and 1999 as shown in Table 7–1.

Net working capital for this simple firm is

NWC = Inventory + Accounts Receivable − Accounts Payable.

For 1999, this figure is 50 + 25 − 30 = $45. This means that the firm has a total of 50 + 25 = $75 worth of short-term assets. Fifty dollars of these assets are inventory, and $25 of these assets is money that is owed to the firm, but hasn't yet been paid, in essence a loan from the firm to its customers. The accounts payable figure of $30 means that the firm owes its suppliers this much, in essence a loan from the suppliers. So the total NWC figure in 1999 of $45 means that the firm has a total of $45 of its own money invested in these short term assets.

The significance of net working capital is not so much the level in a given year, but the changes from year to year. In 1998, net working capital was 45 + 20 − 23 = $42. The increase in NWC of $3 from 1998 to 1999 occurred because the firm grew and found that it had to increase its inven-

Table 7–1 Assets and Liabilites for a Firm

Assets	1999	1998
Inventory	50	45
Accounts Receivable	25	20
Net Plant and Equipment	100	100
Total Assets	175	165
Liabilities		
Accounts Payable	30	23
Debt	60	60
Equity	85	82
Total Liabilities and Equity	175	165

tory by $5 to support the added sales. Since the firm was selling more, it offered more sales on credit, which drove up its accounts receivable by $5 for a total of $10 in new short term assets. However, since the firm was purchasing so many supplies on credit, its accounts payable increased by $7, in effect borrowing an additional $7 from its suppliers in 1999, for an increase in NWC of $3. The significance of this $3 increase in NWC is that it is a genuine investment, it requires actual cash to fund, and occurred as a direct result of the firm's growth. Firms that plan for equipment and plant expansion, but do not plan for investments in net working capital, will find themselves chronically short of cash even though they remain profitable. Interestingly, this problem will become worse, rather than better, if the firm is more successful and grows faster than anticipated.

Free Cash Flow

Free cash flow (FCF) is the money left over after all non-financing expenses have been paid, and all required investment in the company has been made. It is the total amount of cash available to pay interest and principal on debt, and if the firm is a for-profit concern, then dividends:

$$FCF = \text{Operating cash flow} - \text{Gross investment.}$$

Here gross investment consists of investment in equipment, buildings, etc., and investment in NWC.

Positive free cash flows contribute to the market value of a for-profit company. If these free cash flows are bigger than the interest and principal payments, then the firm can even pay dividends without raising additional capital. The same holds true for a not-for-profit company. If the free cash flows for a not-for-profit company are greater than the scheduled interest and principal payments on the company's debt, then the firm is, by definition, able to operate from year to year without resorting to external funding; it is able to generate enough internal funds to finance its projected growth.

On the other hand, if free cash flows are less than the scheduled interest and principal payments on the debt, then the firm will have to raise external capital in order to function from year to year. Persistent negative free cash flows reduce the market value of a for-profit company, and can destroy the financial viability of a not-for-profit company.

A Cash Flow Example

These concepts can best be illustrated with an example. The Powell Gastroenterology Center is a not-for-profit outpatient treatment facility. It is considering expanding its services by both increasing the number of hours of operation per day and adding another procedure room. The result will be an increase in the capacity for procedures of 35 percent. A market analysis has shown that there is sufficient demand in the region to justify the added procedure capacity, and that it will take about three years for the Center to reach full capacity. Procedures per year are projected to increase by 15% the first year, 10% the second year, and 7% the third year. The addition will cost $270,000. The Center will contribute $20,000 of this from its operations and the remaining $250,000 will be financed with a 10-year interest-only bank loan with annual interest payments of $25,000. A balloon payment of $250,000 will be due when the loan matures in 10 years. In addition to the expansion, the Center requires annual upgrades of its existing facilities that total about $10,000 per year. These upgrades are expected to continue.

The projected revenues and costs for the current year, and the first three years of operation are shown in Table 7–2.

Although the procedures increase in each year, profit drops off substantially in the first year because of the added interest payments and the increased depreciation charge due to the new assets. However it does appear that the firm will remain profitable during the startup phase of the expansion, and so management decides to borrow the money and undertake the expansion. Apparently the expansion will not adversely affect the firm's financial position, and there is even a profit cushion of $31,500 in 1998 to help fund any unforeseen problems. The question is: is this analysis sufficient? The answer is no.

Table 7–3 shows some additional figures from the Center's projected balance sheets and a NWC calculation.

These calculations show that the additional interest payments on the $250,000 loan are not the only cash flows required to support the expansion. Because of the increased number of procedure rooms and procedures, inventory and accounts receivable increase. Accounts payable also increase as a result of the increased procedures, which somewhat offsets the increases in accounts receivable and inventory. However, the total increase in NWC amounts to $24,000 in 1999, $18,400 in 2000, and $14,168 in 2001. Adding in the required capital expenses for upgrades of

Table 7–2 Projected Revenues and Costs

	1998	1999	2000	2001
Revenues	250,000	287,500	316,250	338,388
Costs	212,500	244,375	268,813	287,629
Depreciation	6,000	16,000	16,000	16,000
EBIT	31,500	27,125	31,438	34,758
Interest	0	25,000	25,000	25,000
Profit	31,500	2,125	6,438	9,758

$10,000 per year results in a total investment outlay in 1999 of $34,000. Part of this can be paid for out of operating cash flow once depreciation is added back in, but this source of cash is not enough. A free cash flow calculation (Table 7–4) reveals exactly what will happen under the proposed expansion.

The cash surplus line shows that the Center is in fact sufficiently profitable in 1998 to invest the planned $20,000 in the expansion. However, in subsequent years even though the Center remains profitable, the investment in the expansion is complete, and procedures increase as planned, the additional required investment in equipment upgrades and net working capital drain enough cash to create financial difficulties. Even if the Center retains its surplus in 1998 to fund the deficits in 1999 and 2000, the total cash shortfall by the end of 2000 is $7,500 - 15,875 - 5,962 = -$14,337$, and it is not until the end of the year 2002 that this cash short-

Table 7–3 Additional Figures from the Center's Projected Balance Sheets

	1998	1999	2000	2001
Accounts Receivable	140,000	161,000	177,100	189,497
Inventory	70,000	80,500	88,550	94,748
Accounts Payable	50,000	57,500	63,250	67,678
NWC	160,000	184,000	202,400	216,567
Investment in NWC	0	24,000	18,400	14,167
Expansion Outlay	270,000	0	0	0
Other Investment	10,000	10,000	10,000	10,000
Total Investment	280,000	34,000	28,400	24,167

Table 7–4 A Free Cash Flow Calculation

	1998	1999	2000	2001
EBIT	31,500	27,125	31,438	34,758
Taxes	0	0	0	0
NOPAT	31,500	27,125	31,438	34,758
Depreciation	6,000	16,000	16,000	16,000
Operating Cash Flow	37,500	43,125	47,438	50,758
Total Investment	280,000	34,000	28,400	24,167
Free Cash Flow	-222,500	9,125	19,038	26,591
Debt Payments	0	25,000	25,000	25,000
Loan From Bank	250,000	0	0	0
Cash Surplus (Deficit)	7,500	(15,875)	(5,962)	1,591

fall is erased. A firm cannot operate in a cash deficit (unless it defaults on its payments) so something must be done.

A company facing this situation would have a number of alternatives for dealing with the cash shortfalls in 1999 and 2000 if it happened to have performed a cash flow analysis *before* undertaking the project. One possible solution would be to establish a line of credit against which to borrow during the short years. An even simpler solution, if the bank would allow it, would be to borrow the entire $270,000 in 1998 rather than funding a portion of the expansion internally. This would increase interest expenses in each year by $2,000 due to the larger loan, but would increase the surplus in 1998 to $27,500. This surplus would be just barely enough to fund the deficits in 1999, 2000, and 2001 (The deficit in 2001 would come about because the current projected surplus of $1,591 would be reduced by the added interest expense of $2000.)

A company surprised by an unanticipated cash shortfall has fewer alternatives. Most of the time it will resort to a bank loan, if it can get one. Provided there is no other underlying financial instability, the company will probably be able to get such a loan, but the terms may be less favorable than if the company were not desperate. In the absence of a loan, the firm would have to consider which obligations it could safely delay payment on, and the resulting tension between the firm and its suppliers could damage its ability to receive trade credit in the future. This financial distress may also damage the firm's reputation among its customers—further delaying its recovery. It is important to note that all of these problems with cash flow can occur even in firms that are profitable, successful, and growing.

Cash Flows and Equity

The example above illustrates the importance of projecting cash flows associated with expansion projects. Ignoring cash flow in favor of such accounting measures as profit after tax can result in serious management errors—whether in a for-profit or a not-for-profit organization. As important as this is for all firms however, the financial decisions within a stockholder-owned firm provide an even greater challenge to managers than simply remaining financially viable and keeping out of financial distress. This additional challenge to a for-profit corporation is to use the money entrusted to the organization by the stockholders in its most profitable way. Without going into detail about the theory underlying these concepts, simply note that in today's marketplace the stockholders of average-risk companies expect to earn between 10% and 12% per year on their investments. This means that on average, managers of these companies must find projects in which to invest (such as the expansion project above) that earn at least this rate of return on any internally generated or externally provided equity funds invested in the project. Investing in projects with rates of return lower than this destroys shareholder value and reduces the stock price, while investing in projects with rates of return greater than this increases shareholder value and the stock price.

Although the goal of increasing the stock price as much as possible may seem shortsighted in some industries, it is the only feasible goal for a publicly held corporation. Markets today are efficient and complete enough that the management of a firm that consistently earns sub-par rates of returns on its investments will be ousted by the shareholders and replaced. Financial theory shows that the current price of a share of stock is really an aggregate of all of the cash flows that will accrue to the stockholders out into the future by virtue of owning the share of stock. These cash flows are given in the cash surplus (deficit) line of the Powell example above, and managerial actions that improve these cash flows in a sustainable way will increase the stock price.

CONCLUSION

The changing face of health care in this country has forced companies in the industry to come to terms with consolidation and financial restructuring. Consolidation in the number of providers has come about through acquisitions and mergers, and financial restructuring has been required to provide the ready access to capital to fund these purchases. As internal funds have proven inadequate to supply these capital needs, firms have had to choose between external debt and equity. With either choice, there is an increased need to monitor cash flow within the firm. When debt is used to finance growth, firms lose some of the flexibility to weather financial downturns. Firms must carefully plan to have enough cash on hand to meet scheduled debt payments, otherwise financial distress may damage the firm's viability. When equity is used, firms must ensure that the rate of return on the funds used is sufficiently high to compensate the stockholders. This requires careful forecasting of the costs and benefits of projects by specifically projecting their cash flows before the investment is undertaken. The more rapid the growth within a firm, the more important these requirements are.

GLOSSARY

asset. something the company owns or money the company is owed.

collateral. an asset pledged as security on a loan. It may be claimed by the lender if the borrower defaults on the loan.

common stock. the certificate that conveys ownership of a corporation.

debt. bank loans, bond issues, and lines of credit.

debtholder. a lender, or someone who owns a company's bonds.

default. when a borrower misses interest or principal payments on a loan.

depreciation. a line item expense on the income statement that reflects how much a company has "used up" its fixed assets during the year.

equity. a residual claim on profits. This is an ownership claim on the firm.

external capital. debt or equity capital.

free cash flow (FCF). money left over in the company after all non-financing expenses have been paid, and all required investment in the company has been made. FCF = Operating cash flow − Gross investment.

internal capital. investment capital that a company generates from revenues in excess of operating expenses.

liability. money the company owes.

net operating profit after taxes (NOPAT). NOPAT is defined as earnings before interest and taxes (EBIT) less the taxes on EBIT.

net working capital. the difference between short-term assets and short-term liabilities.

non-cash expenses. an expense that appears on the income statement, but does not require a cash payment.

operating cash flow. NOPAT plus non-cash expenses (like depreciation).

private corporation. a corporation whose stock does not trade in the public market.

public corporation. a corporation whose common stock trades on the open market.

restructure. in the context of a loan. The lender postpones interest payments, or reduces the interest rate on the loan, or takes an equity position in exchange for the debt.

secured loan. a loan in which the borrower pledges an asset as collateral.

stockholder. the legal owner of a corporation.

unsecured loan. a loan that does not have specific collateral associated with it.

REFERENCES

Brigham, E.F., Gapenski, L., & Daves, P. (1998). *Intermediate Financial Management*. Fort Worth, TX: The Dryden Press.

CHAPTER 8

Designing, Managing, and Improving Health Care Operations

Charles E. Noon

TABLE OF CONTENTS

EXECUTIVE SUMMARY

The management of business operations encompasses decisions concerning facilities, equipment, materials, personnel, and processes. Taken together, these decisions define the most important function of an organization, the value creation process. The study of business operations is an essential ingredient of an executive MBA program and is especially timely in the context of health care. Under increasing competitive and market pressures, health care providers are discovering that a steady focus on operational excellence is necessary to survive and thrive in the unfolding health care arena.

This chapter discusses the importance of an operations focus and identifies the similarities and differences between health care operations and other types of business operations. An appreciation of these distinctions is an important first step in understanding the applicability and limitations of traditional approaches for the design, management, and improvement of operations. With this knowledge, the challenge for the physician leader is to re-examine familiar systems and processes from a new perspective and to lead organizations towards the goal of providing higher quality health care in a more cost-effective manner.

OPERATIONS AS A TRANSFORMATION PROCESS

In this chapter, we'll be discussing *operations*. Instead of the surgical kind of operations most physicians are familiar with, our focus will be on *business* operations. We can define business operations as the systems and resources that enable a *transformation process*. The classic view of the transformation process is that of inputs passing through an operation, whereby the inputs undergo a transformation and thus emerge as outputs. See Figure 8–1.

The transformation can be *physical.* For example, a paper company has inputs in the form of logs, water, and chemicals. Through its operations consisting of machines, workers, and systems, it *physically* transforms the raw materials into paper. Of course, physical transformation is just one type of a business operation. Airlines provide a *locational* transformation by moving people and cargo. Retail stores facilitate an *exchange* transformation by providing items for sale to customers.

What about the business of health care? If a patient enters an ER with a broken arm and emerges with the arm properly re-set and in a cast, the pa-

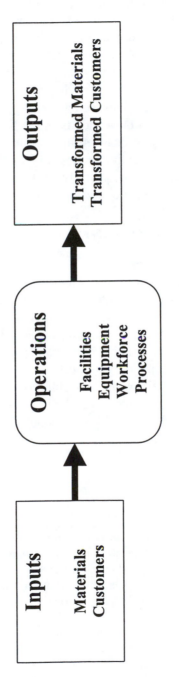

Figure 8–1 Transformation Process

155

tient has undergone a *physiological* transformation. That's easy, but what about the annual check-up patient who is told that an elevated cholesterol level necessitates a change in eating habits? In this case, the health care operation has provided an *informational* transformation process whereby the patient is not transformed physically, but rather emerges from the experience better informed and ultimately healthier.

The management of operations, often referred to as *Operations Management*, encompasses decisions concerning facilities, equipment, materials, personnel, and processes, as given in Exhibit 8–1. Together these elements facilitate the transformation process of a business operation. But as we'll see in this chapter, the business of health care has a number of special characteristics that make it unique and challenging.

ARE OPERATIONS IMPORTANT?

Whether the transformation process is physical, physiological, or informational, it is through *operations* that the actual value is created that the customer is willing to pay for. Without operations, no value is created and a business will cease to be a going concern. Given that, most professionals would agree it should be given *some* managerial attention. Unfortunately, the prevailing attitude about operations has not been to pursue excellence, but rather to avoid doing it poorly.

That was the attitude held by the U.S. automobile manufacturers during the mid-seventies. What unfolded over the next two decades was that the U.S. automakers learned a painful lesson about the importance of opera-

---

Exhibit 8–1 Operational Decisions

Operational Area	Types of Decisions
Facilities	size, layout, location, function
Equipment	type, size, flexibility, quantity
Materials	specifications, vendor relationships, inventory management, material handling
Personnel	qualifications, training, staffing levels, schedule, incentivization
Processes	information flow, customer or product flow, material flow, control

tions and its alignment with customer values. The Big Three mistakenly assumed customers wanted one thing when they really wanted another. They thought consumers wanted large cars with high-priced options and would accept shoddy overall quality. As history shows, the consumers really wanted smaller cars that were simple, low cost, and highly reliable. After some early denial and a couple of years of losing market share, the U.S. automakers finally understood the true values of the customer. However, changing the operations so that they could effectively and profitably deliver those values proved to be a much more arduous task. The final price tag for the Big Three having taken their eyes off of the importance of operations was a major loss of market share accompanied by two decades of gut-wrenching change. To this day, the U.S. firms have never recaptured lost market share and they continue to play catch-up in many areas of automobile design and manufacturing.

The lessons learned from this saga are that businesses cannot market and finance their way to long term sustainability. Finance provides the means to establish operations and marketing creates the demand for the products or services. But ultimately, it is *operations* that must create and deliver the value for which the customer is willing to pay. In the automobile industry, the Japanese were first to discover that operating capabilities can be a primary source of competitive advantage and one that can be difficult and slow to replicate. Hence, a steady focus on Operations not only differentiates you from your competition, but it is something that competitors will be hard pressed to copy and implement. At the same time, however, operations should not be thought of as a function in isolation.

The design and management of operations must work hand-in-hand with the marketing and finance sides of the organization. Marketing establishes the expectations that the service delivery system must ultimately meet. Promises of "eyeglasses in one hour" or "15-minute mortgage approvals" can only be made if they are backed up by a well-designed and managed operation. The marketing department must work to understand the needs and values of customers and to provide information back to the operations managers, who must continually refine the service delivery system. But it is not just a one-directional flow of information. When new operational opportunities or capabilities are discovered at the operating unit level, they must be relayed back to marketing. For example, new techniques and technologies have enabled many conditions to be performed as day surgery rather than in-patient surgery. These advances are then aggressively marketed in order to differentiate health care providers.

WHY DOES A PHYSICIAN LEADER NEED TO KNOW ABOUT OPERATIONS?

Like trying to stand upon shifting ice plates, managing in the health care industry is difficult and challenging. The environment for making business decisions is loaded with uncertainties in the form of ownership, risk, regulations, and technology (Coile, 1997). As we look to the future, however, there are two important certainties. First, from a "business of health care" standpoint, competition will increase and with it will come increased attention to operational costs and quality. Second, with the advancement of "customer choice" in health care, we will witness a continued rise in patient expectations for shorter waits, error-free treatment, and lower costs (Herzlinger, 1997). The good news in all of this is that a goal of providing efficient and high quality health care will apply under any eventual industry landscape that is realized. In other words, operations excellence is probably the only static target in health care today. It is also worth remembering that there is a moral obligation to pursue excellence in operations. There was a time when the poor could not afford shoes due to the high costs associated with shoe production being a craft industry. A consequence of the productivity gains in the shoe industry is that there are more shoes on the feet of the poor. Gains in the efficiency and quality of health care will ultimately help those who cannot afford it and perhaps need it the most.

A better understanding of operations can help a physician leader to navigate through the ever-changing inter-organizational relationships brought about by alliances, mergers, and acquisitions (Rakich, Longest, & Darr, 1992). The motivations behind such actions are often the potential operational gains achievable through the elimination of redundancies and through economies of scale. In negotiating such relationships, the identified gains become the pie, but how the pie is divvied up is often a function of the operational knowledge of the respective parties. This means participants must have not only a profound understanding of their own operations and how they could benefit from a change in relationship, but must be able to quickly understand and assess the operational benefits to be gained by others.

The accelerating rate of change in health care markets, organizations, and technologies requires a physician leader to stay abreast of current operational performance and continuously search for opportunities for improvement. As articulated by Upton (1997), "...the old view of operations management, as the task of running and maintaining a comparatively static production or service facility, has given way to one characterized by a need for renewed flexibility, relentless improvement, and the development of new capabilities at the operating unit level." Just as products have an ever-shrinking life cycle, processes now must be redesigned on a more frequent basis. Information technology is playing a key role towards achieving improved efficiencies, implementing sound business processes, and integrating disparate systems. But rather than locking organizations into static direction or operation, information technology can be implemented in a way that dramatically lowers an organization's barriers to change. In effect, properly designed information systems can allow the organization to be well positioned for operational change and improvement.

If you agree that *operations* are vital to your organization, why not just hire a cadre of experts to make operational decisions for you? First, no outsider can understand your operations like you and your staff. Second, operations improvement is not a one-time endeavor. It is an ongoing process that must be designed into your organization. Third, outside experts are more likely to gravitate towards either the tried-and-true conventional approaches or the current *program-of-the-month*. In doing so, you may be limiting yourself to mediocrity and are more likely to miss opportunities whereby a small innovation due to out-of-the-box thinking might result in tremendous gains.

DESIGNING, MANAGING, AND IMPROVING OPERATIONS

The physician leader must gain an understanding of the concepts of *designing, managing*, and *improving* operations. Operations *design* can be thought of as including all of the things that must be in place before the doors open. Beyond bricks and mortar, it includes equipment, information systems, staffing levels, process flows, and incentive systems. Design also includes decisions related to the scale and scope of an operation. This means the knowledge and understanding of what an operation is capable of doing efficiently and, perhaps more importantly, what it is *not* capable of doing efficiently. In health care, for example, many standard surgical procedures (such as cataract, hernias, etc . . .) are handled very efficiently through focused facilities. System inefficiencies occur when such centers try to take on more general procedures or when hospitals try to run standard procedures through their general surgical process. Design is often under-emphasized yet usually determines the ultimate success of an operation. The best efforts of workers and management cannot overcome a fundamentally bad design.

The concept of *managing* service operations includes all of the activities that ensue once the doors are open. In essence, it is those activities that cannot be designed into the operation beforehand. Examples include identifying and utilizing information about operational performance, market environment, and competition. Managing the balance between demand and resources, managing the workforce, and even short term issues like staff scheduling and dealing with unpredictable events are also included.

Improving operations is about *changing* the design *and* the management of the operation. An axiom of business is that you cannot improve what you don't truly understand. Proper managing of operational information is a must. Another axiom is that it is difficult to improve an operation that was not designed with a goal of *facilitating improvement*. In other words, some operations are robust in that their design recognizes the eventual need for change. By their nature, some managers (and physician leaders) have trouble accepting that they cannot predict the future. Failing to do so can result in an operation that works quite well for a particular health care industry landscape, and quite poorly for any other.

CHARACTERISTICS OF SERVICE OPERATIONS

We distinguish business operations as being either a *goods-producing operation*, such as paper manufacturing, or as a *service operation*, such as a movie theater or a doctor's office. Although we often think about operations management in the context of manufacturing, over 70% of the country's employment is in the form of providing services rather than the manufacturing of goods (Schmenner, 1995). As compared to goods-producing operations, service operations have a number of special challenges. These distinctions limit the extent to which well-studied manufacturing management techniques can be applied to service operations.

High degree of customer interaction with the process

It is likely that few people would know or even care where and how the paper of this book is manufactured. Yet anyone who has visited a bank, restaurant, or retail store, has witnessed the value-creation process firsthand. Not only do customers observe the service delivery operation, they often consider themselves to be experts on them and, if given the chance, will be vigilant in finding operational problems. For example, if you sit down at a restaurant and your service is slow, you are more likely to observe when someone comes in after you but is served before you. The same thing applies to a patient who notices herself and several other 8:00 AM appointments all waiting for the same physician.

Customer demands are mostly immediate

In most service operations, needs must be met in near real-time. A hungry restaurant patron enters an establishment not for a meal to be created and served next week, but rather in the next few minutes. This means careful attention must be given in the capacity design of a service operation. Emergency rooms, for example, must be designed and staffed for a wide range of demand levels and resource requirements.

No equivalent of inventory

Whereas goods-producing operations can build inventories in periods of slack demand, service operations usually cannot. Hotel rooms that are empty on a Wednesday night cannot be used to satisfy a demand that exceeds capacity on the following Saturday night. The same goes for unused block surgery time, unused hospital beds and equipment, and on-call emergency staff during a slow night.

Service quality is difficult to define and measure

In the manufacturing of goods, quality can usually be defined by specifying physical characteristics such as dimension, color, finish, strength, or function. In service operations, defining quality is not so straightforward or objective. The *quality* of a service encounter with an auto repair operation may have less to do with the actual quality of the repair work and more to do with how the customer is treated, the length of wait, the perceived value of the service, and the environment of the facility. This concept is of extreme importance in the business of health care where there has been a mistaken tendency to assume that patients choose providers exclusively on the basis of the quality of patient care, rather than on the overall service experience. As many providers and health care administrators are discovering, that mistake is proving to be very costly.

The definition of service quality differs from person-to-person

A business traveler's evaluation of hotel quality will likely depend on how well the accommodations facilitate the main purpose of the trip, to *work*. The systems and layout that satisfy my definition of quality must coexist with other customers who might be enjoying a vacation and who have a much different set of needs and definition of quality. In health care, one patient may value a physician who spends a lot of time personally interacting while the next may want to spend as little time as possible in getting treated.

Difficulty in separating value-added versus non-value-added activities

When analyzing operations, it is useful to think about activities as being value-added or non-value-added. A value-added activity is usually defined as one that makes a difference to the final customer. For example, the operation of painting a fender is clearly a value-added activity in the making of an automobile. After a fender is stamped out of sheet metal, however, activities such as stacking it, moving a load of fenders to the warehouse, storing the fenders, counting and inspecting the inventory of fenders, and moving fenders to final assembly are all considered non-value-added activities. This type of classification is useful in targeting activities for elimination or improvement. In service operations, the distinctions are less obvious. For example, suppose patients are given a reminder phone call the day before a scheduled appointment. Is that a value-added activity or not?

Service experiences often span multiple areas and organizations

Most service operation processes involve a coordinated sequence of front room and back room activities. In some cases, the full process may involve off-premise activities. In an auto-repair situation, a manager's promise to "get the part in a couple of hours" means the entire process now involves activities that are remote with respect to location and organization. Physician offices usually send out lab work and, in some cases, will even route the patients to other facilities for tests.

SPECIAL CHALLENGES WITHIN HEALTH CARE SERVICE OPERATIONS

Health Care in the Context of Service Operations

Health care has particular characteristics that distinguish it from other service operations. Some of these distinctions are due to the nature of health care and some are due to the industry's emerging transition from its not-for-profit origins.

Health care transformation processes are broad in scope and duration

A hungry individual may choose to go into a restaurant and enjoy a meal. When finished, the check is paid and the entire service encounter is complete. In health care, the transformation process can range from a simple one-time visit to one of numerous visits spanning a longstanding relationship. For example, a one-time encounter might be a visit to an ambulatory treatment center to treat a minor medical emergency. In contrast, the treatment for a condition such as diabetes will span years and may involve a number of medical stages and providers. Setting up service operations to efficiently deliver at both extremes is quite difficult.

Health care transformation processes can be reactive or proactive

Most people take their car in for service when they decide it is time for maintenance (according to the manual) or when there is a problem that needs fixing. Many decisions to seek health care are made in a similar fashion. In contrast, a dentist might keep track of a patient's last visit and call the patient when it has been about six months since a prior visit. Any problems are caught very early and can be treated in a low cost (and low pain) fashion. From a business standpoint, this practice provides the dentist with a steady, predictable stream of low-margin business activity. Without the proactive contact, the patient's dental needs would more likely consist of a collection of episodic high-margin acute dental care to treat festered problems. In essence, the dentist is moving patient demands on the system from totally random to somewhat predictable. From an operations perspective, there is often value in doing so.

Health care services are complex

Many medical services involve a relatively wide array of people, equipment, materials, and processes. Take, for instance, a typical surgery department. In order to accomplish a surgical procedure, a large number of individuals must be involved either directly or indirectly including anesthesiologist, surgeon, orderlies, RNs, clerks, materials managers, equipment providers, pharmacy personnel, tray assemblers, housekeeping, and many others. The individuals differ considerably with respect to wages, incentives, and even employment. Add to that the different types of equipment that must be in proper working order and the surgical trays that must be correctly picked ahead of time. All materials, pharmaceuticals, and supplies must be available in inventory. And finally, the processes and sequences of task and approvals must be defined for and understood by all involved personnel and then executed flawlessly. In terms of complexity and coordination, a surgical procedure is more like making an airline flight happen than simply fixing a car. And that's just the take-off. Look beyond the surgical procedure both forward and backward in time and you'll see a process that is multi-staged and whose coordination is driven by information.

Health care operations are expensive relative to most service operations

It involves expensive materials, expensive equipment, and expensive personnel. That effectively guarantees that any inefficiencies or redundancies will always be costly.

Customers are often only indirectly responsible for paying for the service

Another aspect that distinguishes health care operations from most service operations is that the customer receiving the value is often only indirectly responsible for paying for the service. The environment, depending on whether it is one of managed care, capitation, or fee-for-service, will dramatically affect both the customer and the service provider.

There is considerable variation in customer needs and provider practices

Customers differ with respect to their health care needs. Some of the variation is due to physiological differences and some is due to individual preferences. On the provider side, the system resources required in treating a patient exhibit considerable variation as well. The practice of medicine is still considered an art and many physicians are inherently resistant to attempts at reducing variation through systemization.

Emotional issues

Like no other "business," the transformation processes of health care deals with the life and death of people. Any operational decision carries with it some effect on patient safety and quality of treatment. Trust plays an important role in the customer-provider relationship and is an element that is difficult, if not impossible, to measure in the classic view of operations management.

Incentives may not be clear or well aligned

It's no secret that incentives and measures will drive behavior in the workplace. Often problems that appear to be operational in nature turn out to be caused by the incentive structure designed into the system. Detecting such problems in health care is complicated by the fact that most health care workers are largely driven by the well-being of patients. This results in situations where workers will make things work in spite of a poor incentive or operational design. The need to look closely at behavioral drivers becomes even more challenging as incentives become relatively less direct within the strategies of managed care, risk distribution, and capitation.

The Phenomenon of Queuing

The concept of queuing is best illustrated through the use of an example. Let's suppose you are the only physician on staff at a walk-in clinic. Let's also assume that a patient walks in the door *precisely* every 20 minutes and it takes you *exactly* 15 minutes to treat a patient. Your day is a repeating cycle of treat for 15, idle for 5, treat for 15, idle for 5, and so on. Your utilization (the percent of time you are busy) is 75%. Each patient arrives, has no wait, and is treated in 15 minutes. This scenario sounds too good to be true and is a far cry from reality.

Let's modify it to be more realistic. Let's say, instead, that you get *on average* three patient arrivals per hour or 1 patient per 20 minutes. They arrive not in a pattern of uniform intervals, but rather in the kind of unpredictable fashion you would expect in a walk-in environment. And rather than precise treatment times, let's assume that the time it takes to treat a patient *averages* 15 minutes, but it can range from just several minutes to more than an hour depending on the condition of the patient. Although you will still have an average utilization of 75% in this scenario, your day will no longer be a predictable, repeating cycle of treating time and idle. You and the patients will have much different experiences than in the earlier version. In fact, patients will wait before starting treatment an average of *45 minutes*. Their individual waiting times will range from zero to more than an hour or two. On average, there will be *3 patients* in the clinic either being treated or·waiting to be treated. As the physician, you will go through long periods of treating patients in a non-stop fashion and at other times you may have periods of no patients at all. Over the course of a week, some days will be hectic and others will be easy. Does this sound more realistic?

The system is behaving according to the laws of queuing. The queuing phenomenon is well studied both theoretically and empirically. Any service operation that has randomly generated demands and variable service times will have some degree of queuing. For this same example, let's now suppose that due to some new marketing efforts, the rate of patient arrivals increases slightly to the point where a patient arrives every 17 minutes on average. In this case, your utilization will increase to a respectable 88.2% (15 divided by 17), but what happens to the queue? Patient waits before treatment will average 112.5 minutes and there will be an average of 7.5 patients in the clinic either being treated or waiting. For this *single-server queue model*, we can plot the average pre-treatment waiting times and the expected number of patients in the clinic as a function of utilization (see Figures 8–2 and 8–3). As we push up the utilization, the queue statistics grow considerably worse.

Any time that a call for service is generated randomly from a population, some degree of queuing for the server will ensue. Queuing situations abound in health care as there is no way we can predict when symptoms will present or when accidents will occur. The obvious examples are walk-in services and calls for appointments to a doctor's office. Less obvious queuing situations arise without the actual telltale waiting line. For example, in-patient calls to a nursing station or calls to orderly and housekeeping pools all occur in a random fashion. As a result, classic "efficiency-based" approaches to managing in health care operations must be applied with considerable caution. In addition, we can make the observation that some degree of waiting is inevitable in such systems.

There are a number of strategies that an operations manager can pursue in trying to dealing with the phenomenon of queuing. These include trying to influence the demand side, trying to improve capacity management on the resource side, trying to remove randomness from the server operation, and as a last resort trying to affect the customer's perception of waiting. Regarding the latter, it was discovered long ago in the hotel industry that complaints of slow elevators can be virtually eliminated by flanking elevators with full-length mirrors. By doing so, an empty wait for an elevator is turned into productive opportunity to complete one's grooming process (i.e., *primp*). In health care systems, the use of cross-trained staff, coordinated operating room scheduling, and pooled resources are all ways to help combat the effects of queuing.

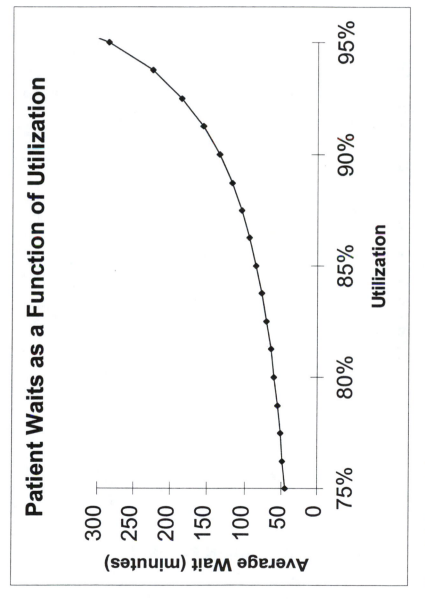

Figure 8-2 Patient Waiting Times

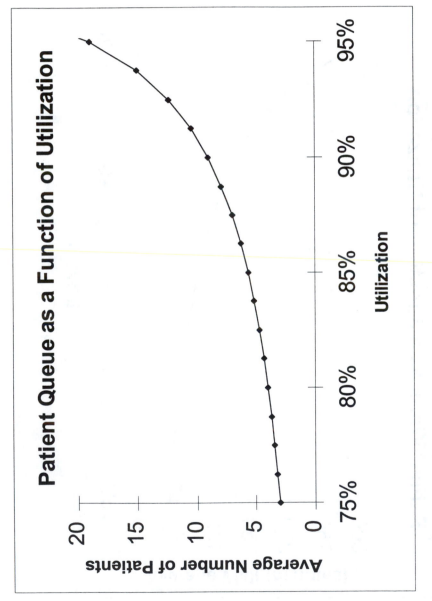

Figure 8–3 Patient Queue Lengths

Interdependent Activities and Variation

A physician leader must develop a sharp eye for sources of variation and must understand how variation affects health care operations. *Variation* is the extent to which a process differs from the norm (Deming, 1986; McLaughlin & Kaluzny, 1994). In general, operational performance deteriorates when high levels of variation occur within processes that have a high degree of interdependency. The problem symptoms are poor capacity usage, shifting bottlenecks, and excessive waits. There are plenty of health care examples of sequential, interdependent activities such as a patient flow through pre-op, surgery and recovery, or an office visit with X-rays, lab work, and examination. In these cases, the sequential activities are highly *interdependent* since an activity must not only succeed another, but in some cases must follow closely in time. Interdependent activities are not necessarily a problem, but in the presence of *variation,* such processes become very difficult to manage efficiently. Keep in mind that, in sequential processes, variation is additive and does not cancel itself out. The childhood "telephone game" was actually a lesson in compound variation within a sequential process.

The notion of interdependent activities with variation is not something new. Goods-producing operations have always had interdependent activities with variation but they have traditionally (and incorrectly) relied on inventory as an "accommodating" buffer between interdependent activities. Take, for example, a part that is produced and then used in a subsequent assembly operation. If there was variation in the quantity of nondefective parts in a production run, then a manager could play it safe by building up a sizable inventory between the production of the part and the part's subsequent operation. Without the option of inventory, the need for zero defects and variation reduction within service operations is even more critical. There are plenty of sources of arguably *inherent* or *unpreventable* variation in health care such as variation in the severity of a condition or variation in patient responses to treatment. Too often, however, health care professionals are quick to assume *preventable* variation is just part of the business.

Recall that in queuing systems with truly random demands, a system behaves in an unpredictable fashion, thus making it very difficult for which to plan. In many health care processes, interdependent activities are often "informationally" disconnected, which effectively turns predictable demands into random demands and brings about operational difficulties.

For example, a surgery department will prepare for a scheduled appendectomy only to find out at the time of surgery that the patient has *known* complicating conditions (obesity, diabetes) that were not communicated and which will alter the equipment needs and lengthen the procedure. This, in turn, sets off a scramble for equipment and results in delayed start times for later procedures. Had the staff been advised of the known conditions, it would have been able to anticipate the equipment needs and longer procedure time. This example illustrates the problems caused by preventable (or at least, reducible) variation that is assumed to be unpreventable or inherent to healthcare. Variation reduction in health care can often be achieved by recognizing the sources and applying efficient information linkages and developing the ability to properly utilize the information.

Systems Within Systems

The hardest thing to do when you are working in a system is to work on the system. In fact, who has the time or inclination to even *look* at the system much less try to fix it? An important skill for physician leaders is the ability to raise their perspective "up a level" when systemic problem symptoms present. A hospital is a system that is usually organized and managed in departmental fashion. A department manager focuses mainly on local optimization within the measures established for the department. We tend to admire and praise the fire-fighting supervisor who can always get through the daily crisis imposed upon his or her department by the system. But chronic operational fire fighting should be recognized for what it is, a clear symptom of problems at the systems level.

Departments greatly influence each other's operational performance and, taken together, they ultimately define the experience of the customer. Think of how the responsiveness and error rate of an ancillary service (like the lab) can affect a department and ultimately the customer. But the question is who is looking at and working on the hospital as a *system*? Who truly understands the interdependencies and processes of the whole system? The answer is probably no one person. It requires a conscious, collective team-based effort.

The value of gaining a systems perspective extends far beyond helping to solve *problems* that can't be solved at the local level. It is often the systems that appear to be "problem-less" that offer the greatest opportunities for removing system costs and increasing quality. The medical products supply chain is a good example where opportunities for systems improvement exist at the inter-organizational level. Think of the costs that a hospital must incur to purchase, receive, and manage inventories of materials. Think also of the costs that a distributor must incur to fulfill orders, ship, and manage inventories of materials. Now imagine how much of the costs could be removed if the goal between the organizations was to streamline the purchaser-supplier activities and reduce the total system inventories. Take that a step further and envision the same goals applied throughout the medical products supply chain spanning from manufacturer to end-user. A recent study examined that particular issue and estimated that $11 billion (48%) of the $23 billion in supply chain *process* costs are avoidable in the existing health care products supply chain (Efficient Healthcare Consumer Response [EHCR], 1996). Such gains are possible only through the attainment of a systems perspective and a coordinated inter-organizational effort.

Keep in mind also that systems are nested. A department is a system within a hospital, a hospital is a system within a network, a network is a system within the health care industry, and the health care industry is a system within the overall economy. Gaining a systems perspective is sort of like scaling a mountain. As soon as you gain a higher perspective, it's time to start looking even higher.

CONCLUSION

The successful physician leader must be equipped with a solid understanding of the value-creation process. Relative to many other service operations, health care delivery systems have some characteristics that make it similar and some that make it distinct. The challenge for the physician leader is to re-examine familiar systems and processes in a new light and to use this new perspective to lead organizations towards providing higher quality health care in a more cost-effective manner.

GLOSSARY

goods-producing operation. a business operation whereby the output of the transformation process is a tangible good.

operations management. the management of decisions that concern facilities, equipment, materials, personnel, and processes.

queuing. the emergence of a waiting line when random arrivals generate demands on a finite-capacity server.

service operation. a business operation whereby no tangible good is produced.

transformation process. inputs transformed into outputs as facilitated by business operations.

variation. the extent to which a process differs from the norm.

REFERENCES

Coile, R. (1997). *The five stages of managed care: Strategies for providers, HMOs, and suppliers*. Ann Arbor, MI: Health Administration Press.

Deming, W. (1986). *Out of the crisis*. Cambridge, MA: MIT Center for Advanced Engineering Study.

EHCR. (1996). *Efficient Healthcare Consumer Response (EHCR), improving the efficiency of the healthcare supply chain*. Alexandria, VA: CSC Consulting.

Herzlinger, R. (1997). *Market driven health care: Who wins, who loses in the transformation of America's largest service industry*. Reading, MA: Addison-Wesley Publishing Co.

McLaughlin, C., & Kaluzny, A. (1994). *Continuous quality improvement in health care*. Gaithersburg, MD: Aspen Publishers.

Rakich, J., Longest, B., & Darr, K. (1992). *Managing health services organizations* (3rd ed.). Baltimore: Health Professions Press.

Schmenner, R. (1995). *Service operations management*. Englewood Cliffs, NJ: Prentice Hall.

Upton, D. (1997). *Designing, managing and improving operations processes* (HBSP case note 5-697-065). Cambridge, MA: Harvard Business School Press.

CHAPTER 9

Disease Management: What Every Physician Leader Needs to Know

Donald E. Lighter

TABLE OF CONTENTS

EXECUTIVE SUMMARY

Disease management describes a process that should seem familiar to most physician leaders, but actually it subsumes a process that transcends direct patient care and deals with disease entities and interventions in populations. The processes of disease management include tools such as evaluating the disease burden of a population, stratifying the population into intervention groups, and then various interventions from preventive education to intense case management. Because of the need for an understanding of disease processes and therapies, physician leaders can contribute immeasurably to the creation and implementation of disease management programs. Most physicians, however, lack training in population analysis, which is a skill critical to effectively implementing a disease management program. Physician leaders who have achieved the distinction of a Masters degree in Business Administration must be facile with the disease management paradigm; thus, a substantial portion of the curriculum of a physician-oriented MBA program must be devoted to disease management and its closely associated subject of continuous quality improvement.

THE CONCEPT AND RATIONALE OF DISEASE/CARE MANAGEMENT

Paraphrasing W. Edwards Deming, one of the most overstated realities in health care today is one which physicians readily acknowledge, i.e. change isn't coming, it's happening now. Mid-career practitioners are often alarmed and dismayed by the changes in health care that are occurring, often without their input, but there are a number of new trends that provide hope for health practitioners. Disease Management, or Care Management as many health care managers prefer, promises to help improve the quality of patient care, while helping remove the burden of nonmedical patient management activities from the physician's shoulders. Fortunately, care management requires physician input and participation to succeed, and the process results in improved patient care, decreased payer and provider costs, and enhanced provider and patient satisfaction with the outcomes of health care.

In the course of analyzing patterns of care for their high cost members, managed care organizations (MCOs) discovered problems with current practices of caring for patients with chronic disorders. Duplicated services, adverse drug interactions, and overuse of some unnecessary or inappropriate services were accompanied by failure of patients to seek care from appropriate providers or failure of providers to coordinate patient care. For example, the use of beta-blockers after myocardial infarction is well established medical practice, but in some areas of the country, only 15% of patients receive this important therapy (National Committee on Quality Assurance [NCQA], 1997). Similarly, childhood immunization rates remain abysmally low in spite of the clear efficacy of immunizations in preventing serious childhood illnesses (NCQA, 1997). On the other hand, rates of some interventions, e.g. Caesarean sections, remain excessively high (NCQA, 1997). These problems, combined with the high cost and growth in expenditures of medical care in the 1980s and 1990s, led MCOs to implement cost containment programs, designed to reduce the cost of care received by their members by reducing the burden of inappropriate care. Physicians often complained about the excessive administrative burden that emanated from these programs, and MCOs were continually beset by providers' efforts to circumvent these unwanted authoritarian intrusions. Disease management evolved as one method by which physicians and MCOs can work together, using the strengths of each, to simultaneously lower costs and improve patient care.

Most physicians are familiar with the interventions of MCOs to cut costs by denying inappropriate care or reducing the level of care, but many providers have only recently recognized the benefits of care management as a means of reducing costs. By increasing patient access to preventive care and by expediting needed care, patient health can be improved, leading to greater wellness and lower costs. Such an approach requires greater levels of MCO cooperation with providers, both for defining appropriate care and for improving patient compliance. Thus, many physicians are now forming new partnerships with payers, rather than perpetuating the traditional adversarial relationships.

Care management evolved from the cost containment programs used by MCOs in the 1980s and 1990s. Numerous publications have demonstrated that the cost of caring for chronic conditions consumed a large portion of health expenditures (Flaum, Lung, & Tinkelman, 1997; Hanchak, 1995; Lucas, Gunter, Byrnes, Coyle, & Friedman, 1995), and so disease management programs have assumed increasing importance in targeting those conditions for intervention. Insurers have rapidly recognized, however, that disease management programs could not succeed without physician input and cooperation. Complex patients require substantial amounts of time and expertise for appropriate management, and physicians provide the key knowledge base of diagnosis and treatment required for effective programs. Physicians frequently absorb the cost of non-clinical activities, e.g. obtaining prior authorization for services, scheduling procedures, and insuring that non-clinical resources like transportation are available for their patients, areas in which MCOs have gained experience in the past few years. Thus, a synergism existed to create an effective partnership.

COMPONENT CARE: THE FAILED MODEL

To make these relationships succeed, payers and providers are starting to abandon the costly and inefficient methods of component care, i.e. disease-focused acute care with reimbursement skewed toward procedures and acute exacerbations of underlying disease processes. This outmoded approach to care was a natural outgrowth of health care research in the twentieth century, which emphasized increasing specialization to successfully apply the fruits of medical research. Physicians were encouraged through training programs and reimbursement patterns to become more specialized in order to better serve the patient population. The net result of this evolution in medical practice has been fragmentation of patient care, leading to some of the problems previously mentioned. In a component care system, patients receive services from a variety of physicians and other providers, with little coordination of care and frequent conflicts or duplications in diagnostic and therapeutic modalities. Unfortunately, this duplicative care often caused increased morbidity, leading to greater cost and patient dissatisfaction (Classen, Pestotnik, Evans, Lloyd, & Burke, 1997; Bates et. al., 1997).

Another outgrowth of the component care system is the excessive variation that ensues from failure to coordinate patient care. Errors of omission and commission are common. Providers order duplicate tests because information is either not available or inadequate, or providers fail to order services, assuming that other providers caring for the patient will assume that responsibility. Either course of action increases costs and decreases the quality of patient care, leading to greater consumer dissatisfaction and further incursion by MCOs into medical practice. Health care delivery systems are becoming increasingly integrated in an effort to better coordinate care, but they often find themselves mimicking the MCOs that they eschew so that they can effectively oversee patient care.

As the constraints of the new era of health care economics became manifest in the 1980s, component care approaches proved ineffective in meeting the new financial and marketing challenges of a consumer-driven health care market. Payers perceived lower value for health care expenditures, since the cost of care far exceeded quality, even with the crude quality measurement systems of the 1970s and 1980s. Federal and state governments began funding experimental models of prepaid care for Medicare and Medicaid beneficiaries. Health care consumers (patients) increasingly expressed dissatisfaction with the quality of care. Consumer, governmental, and employer pressure have rapidly produced the changes in the health care delivery system that prevention-oriented physicians have sought for years—increased emphasis on wellness, continuity of care, and physician-patient relationships.

PHARMACEUTICAL COMPANIES: A GROWING FORCE IN DISEASE MANAGEMENT

Pharmaceutical companies have become another preeminent force in the marketplace in the late twentieth century. As MCOs and integrated delivery systems recognized that pharmaceutical costs accounted for huge proportions of health care expenditures, they pushed to encourage providers to prescribe generic drugs, rather than excessively costly trade-name drugs. MCOs and other payers now deal directly with pharmaceutical manufacturers to negotiate discounts and rebates on drugs, often causing large shifts in utilization over relatively short periods of time. Pharmaceutical manufacturers can see the market share for a specific drug change radically in a matter of a few months, wreaking havoc on cash flow, distribution systems, and profit margins. One strategy that the pharmaceutical companies have pursued is the creation or purchase of organizations that perform pharmacy benefit management (PBM). These companies contract with MCOs and providers to attenuate drug use by members, and a common technique employed is the use of disease management programs. The influence of these PBMs has become so pervasive, that most now are subsidiaries of major pharmaceutical companies.

Regardless of which organization in the health care delivery system initiates care management, there are several important attributes of these programs. First, the focus of care management is on prevention and health maintenance, rather than repair and reconstruction. Myriad cost effectiveness studies have demonstrated the benefits of prevention in reducing health care costs (NIH Consensus Panel on Physical Activity and Cardio-vascular Health, 1996), and effective care management programs promote preventive care, as well as continuity of care. Second, financial rewards in the system are not related to the ability to perform esoteric procedures, but rather the reduction in the need for expensive procedures and diagnostic interventions. Prevention of disease now has become as important as treatment of disease, and care management programs ensure that these preventive efforts are rewarded. Importantly, many of the tools of prevention are not clinical (removal of lead–contaminated paint from the dwellings of young children or achievement of high screening rates for breast and cervical cancer) but providers who promote these interventions are gradually being recognized and rewarded for their efforts.

ELEMENTS OF CARE MANAGEMENT

Care management must be differentiated from case management to fully understand its impact. Physicians are accustomed to evaluating patient care at the level of the individual patient, and case management is one of the tools that care managers employ to implement care management programs. Case management entails the skills and techniques for ensuring appropriateness and quality of care for individual patients, usually those with chronic disorders that require substantial coordination of care. Care management, however, refers to the data analysis and interventions for either a disease entity or a preventive health intervention for an entire population. The disease entity or preventive service defines the population, e.g. all diabetics for a diabetes disease management program or all women over forty years of age for a mammography screening program. Case managers, usually experienced nurses, implement the care management program on a case by case basis in the defined population. For example, although the diabetes disease management program may serve all diabetics, only a subset of diabetics may be selected for case management.

THE ROLE OF CASE MANAGEMENT IN DISEASE/CARE MANAGEMENT

Designers of disease management programs must have in-depth knowledge of the characteristics of the problem, including:

- pathophysiology of the disease entity
- effective treatment modalities for the disease entity
- morbidity and mortality associated with treatments
- methods of patient selection for treatment
- demographic profile of the target population
- barriers to access for patients
- areas of deficiency in current patterns of care
- ability to understand statistical analyses of patterns of diagnosis and treatment
- capacity to segment the population into targets for intervention
- provider attitudes and opinions about the disease and treatments
- effective methods of educating providers and patients regarding the disease and treatments
- ability to work in a team environment

KNOWLEDGE BASE FOR CARE MANAGEMENT

Physician leaders are ideal for designing disease management programs, in conjunction with other health professionals, and a thorough understanding of the care management paradigm is necessary for any physician leader. In fact, a substantial amount of time is devoted in a physician-oriented Executive MBA program to insure a thorough understanding of the care management paradigm.

CHARACTERISTICS OF CARE MANAGEMENT ORGANIZATIONS

Organizations that design and implement disease or care management programs must also have certain important characteristics:

- ability to collaborate with providers and other health professionals in a collegial manner
- willingness to fund development activities
- information systems capable of collecting and analyzing complex clinical and administrative data sets
- information systems capable of examining data from patient interactions using the tools developed in the disease management program
- willingness to change reimbursements to encourage preventive care

- staff capable of implementing the interventions recommended by the disease management program designers

MCOs are often ideally suited to develop disease management programs because of their robust information systems, but few have the breadth of resources internally to successfully address all of the issues listed above. Often, MCOs have placed themselves in antagonistic relationships with providers because of the disputes over component care issues, and so they must devote precious time and resources to mending those relationships before mounting effective disease management programs.

Pharmaceutical companies also have powerful information management systems that can perform the analyses necessary for developing effective disease management programs. These organizations frequently have much better relationships with providers, expediting creation of working arrangements. Additionally, the pharmaceutical manufacturers have a vast amount of data on drugs and drug interactions that is critical for effective disease management. However, pharmaceutical companies rarely have much reimbursement data beyond that for pharmaceuticals.

Physicians and other providers possess the invaluable knowledge base of disease diagnosis and treatment to contribute to the disease management development process. Nearly all provider groups lack important resources, like capital and information management systems, to apply the information to effectively create disease management programs. Although many professional medical organizations are working to establish themselves as expert resources for disease management programs, without the critical resources to develop and implement programs, these organizations are often perceived as serving only professional self-interest.

Finally, government could assemble all of the necessary resources, but the current political environment precludes any significant initiatives. After the debacle of the Clinton health plan in the early 1990s, federal and state government officials are reticent to move into a clinical area like disease management, but legislators presently seem to prefer taking smaller steps, like legislatively mandating certain screening programs or treatment modalities. Although this approach is shortsighted and costly, it does impel the health care delivery system to accelerate development of comprehensive disease management programs.

CROSS-INDUSTRY TEAMS

The obvious answer to the conundrum is the creation of cross-industry teams composed of representatives from MCOs, providers, payers, patients, and pharmaceutical companies, all of which can bring a needed set of skills and resources to the process. Physician leaders will be needed to guide these efforts, since they are the only stakeholders that interface directly with all of the other participants in the process. Although clinicians have many of the skills necessary to serve this function, the appropriately trained physician leader will be one with an understanding of disease management, finance, group dynamics, and the legal environment of health care.

THE ROLE OF CLINICAL PRACTICE GUIDELINES IN CARE MANAGEMENT

The disease or care management program will have at its core an evidence-based clinical practice guideline (CPG). The Agency for Health Care Policy and Research (AHCPR) defines a clinical practice guideline as "systematically developed statements to assist practitioners' and patients' decisions about health care to be provided for specific clinical circumstances" (U.S. Department of Health and Human Services, 1995). The important concept underlying clinical practice guidelines is the premise that they are designed to be best practices, rather than reimbursement models. The CPG utilizes published evidence from scientific studies to the greatest extent possible, data from quality improvement studies in affected populations as a secondary resource, and finally consensus among experts in management of a specific disease or preventive modality when other evidence is not available. Importantly, the CPG process relies on scientific data, rather than just consensus.

INTERVENTION TOOLS FOR CARE MANAGEMENT

Once the CPG has been developed, specific intervention tools are developed for case managers and clinicians. Tools for care management vary depending on the target population. Some examples include:

- newsletters and informational mailings to target population on the disease and effective treatments

- telephone hotlines for questions and acute care management
- informational communications to providers regarding the best practices identified in the CPG
- case management and expedited referral processes for high risk patients in the population
- seminars and educational sessions for providers and patients regarding the program
- provider profiles to provide feedback to providers regarding their adherence to best practices
- publication of clinical guidelines on a web site accessible to providers and patients
- financial program redesign, e.g. elimination of copays and deductibles, to encourage compliance with the disease management program
- elimination of need for prior authorization and referral certification for providers who comply with the program

All of these efforts are directed at changing provider and patient behavior to comply with the disease management program. One of the skills of an effective physician leader is the ability to communicate the advantages of the disease management program to providers and patients in a manner that improves compliance (Goldberg et. al., 1998; Soumerai et. al., 1998).

The success of disease management programs relies heavily on continuous data collection and analysis to demonstrate improvement in the care of the population of patients with the disease. With the CPG as the nominal standard of care, provider performance and patient outcomes are continuously measured using sophisticated information systems to insure that the program is effective in improving health. Additionally, experienced disease managers and physician leaders must regularly sift through the medical literature to update the program based on new medical research. As needs for change are identified, the program is modified to reflect the most current evidence-based practice recommendations. Only through this continuous improvement process will the disease management system maintain credibility with providers and patients, and the leadership of physicians versed in methods of quality improvement and care management will be of central importance in guaranteeing the success of these programs.

CONCLUSION

The concept of care management serves as one of the key integrating mechanisms in the new economic environment of health care. Stakeholders in all areas of the health care system, including consumers, have a vested interest in ensuring that these programs succeed, since the quality of care can improve at the same time costs are reduced. Although care management programs require a wealth of resources, cooperation between the participants in the health care delivery system can ensure that adequate intellectual and material assets can be applied to optimize these systems for the benefit of patients. Physician leaders with a thorough understanding of the care management paradigm can be instrumental in leading these efforts.

GLOSSARY

care management. the data analysis and interventions for either a disease entity or a preventive health intervention for an entire population.

clinical practice guideline. systematically developed statements to assist practitioners' and patients' decisions about health care to be provided for specific clinical circumstances.

component care. disease focused acute care geared toward palliating an acute disease process or the acute phase of a chronic disease process.

continuity of care. consistent and carefully supervised health care services designed to enhance the health of the patient; usually supervised by a primary care provider.

disease management. a process of complete integration of prevention, diagnosis, management, and reimbursement based on the natural course of a disease.

integrated delivery system. a health care organization capable of providing virtually all patient care within the organization.

managed care organizations. organizations, e.g. health maintenance organizations and some preferred provider organizations, that contract with payers to supervise patient care in a population.

The National Committee for Quality Assurance (NCQA). a not-for-profit organization created to monitor and accredit managed care organizations.

patterns of care. methods of diagnosis, treatment, and prevention used by practitioners in managing a disease entity or preventive health services for a patient or population of patients.

Pharmacy Benefit Management (PBM). a system for monitoring use of pharmaceuticals and creation of intervention strategies to address aberrant utilization patterns

provider. in the health care industry, a provider is any trained health care professional rendering services to patients.

standard of care. a target practice pattern for a diagnostic or treatment modality.

REFERENCES

Bates, D.W., Spell, N., Cullen, D.J., Burdick, E., Laird, N., Petersen, L.A., Small, S.D., Sweitzer, B.J., & Leape, L.L. (1997). Adverse drug events prevention study group, the costs of adverse drug events in hospitalized patients. *Journal of the American Medical Association, 277,* 307–311.

Classen, D.C., Pestotnik, S.L., Evans, R.S., Lloyd, J.F., & Burke, J.P. (1997). Adverse drug events in hospitalized patients, excess length of stay, extra costs, and attributable mortality. *Journal of the American Medical Association, 277,* 301–306.

Flaum, M., Lung, C.L., & Tinkelman, D. (1997). Take control of high-cost asthma. *Journal of Asthma, 34,* 5.

Goldberg, H.I., Wagner, E.H., Fihn, S.D., Martin, D.P., Horowitz, C.R., Christensen, D.B., Cheadle, A.D., Diehr, P., & Simon, G. (1998). A randomized controlled trial of CQI teams and academic detailing: Can they alter compliance with guidelines? *Journal on Quality Improvement, 24*(3), 130–142.

Hanchak, N.A. (1995) The epidemiology of costs of diabetes mellitus. *US Quality Algorithms, Quality Monitor, 2,* 5.

Lucas, J., Gunter, M.J., Byrnes, J., Coyle, M., & Friedman, N. (1995). Integrating outcomes measurement into clinical practice improvement across the continuum of care: A disease-specific episode of care model. *Managed Care Quarterly, 3,* 14.

National Committee on Quality Assurance. (1997). HEDIS Measures for Managed Care Organizations. Available: http://www.ncqa.org/hedis [1998, June 10].

NIH Consensus Development Panel on Physical Activity and Cardiovascular Health. (1996, July 17). Physical activity and cardiovascular health. *Journal of the American Medical Association, 276,* 241–246.

Soumerai, S.B., McLaughlin, T.J., Gurwitz, J.H., Guadagnoli, E., Hauptman, P.J., Borbas, C., Morris, N., McLaughlin, B., Gao, X., Willison, D.J., Asinger, R., & Gobel, F. (1998). Effect of local medical opinion leaders on quality of care for acute myocardial infarction: A randomized controlled trial. *Journal of the American Medical Association, 279,* 1358–1363.

U. S. Department of Health and Human Services. (1995, March). Using clinical practice guidelines to evaluate quality of care. AHCPR Publication number 95–0045.

PART III

Leading Exemplar Performance

CHAPTER 10

Strategic Leadership in the Health Care Industry

William Q. Judge

TABLE OF CONTENTS

EXECUTIVE SUMMARY

Given the tremendous changes that confront the health care industry in the United States, there is a growing need for strategic leadership on the part of physician executives. Armed with their clinical training and expertise with strategic leadership concepts and skills, physicians can become proactive change makers rather than passive change takers.

This chapter explores the concept of strategic leadership, which is the central focus of my teaching, research, consulting, and health care governance experiences. The concept of leadership is differentiated from the concept of management in an attempt to clarify these two complementary, but distinct practices within organizations. Next, a particular type of leadership, namely strategic leadership, is explored and its importance and impact on organizations is discussed. Finally, the two key dimensions of strategic leadership—competencies and character—are identified and some concepts and details about each are provided.

To address the changing health care industry, creative and effective leadership is needed. This is particularly true of physician leaders who are uniquely positioned to show the way to integrate the clinical and business aspects of the health care delivery system. This chapter discusses some key concepts and skills required by physician leaders that are currently needed in the rapidly evolving health care industry. It begins with a discussion of the author's experience base with the health care industry and proceeds to discuss some of the fundamental ideas that will be necessary for physician leaders to know and master if they desire to assume a leadership role.

MY PERSPECTIVE

I currently serve on the board of directors of St. Mary's Health System, a $150 million, private, non-profit health care delivery system located in East Tennessee. This system is comprised of two acute care hospitals, one long-term rehabilitation facility; a for-profit entity that handles new business ventures and physician practice management services; a growing philanthropic foundation; a PPO network; and several strategic alliances with managed care firms.

St. Mary's is a member of a larger health care delivery system named Catholic Healthcare Partners (CHP). CHP is headquartered in Cincinnati, Ohio, and is currently the sixth-largest health delivery system in the United States. In 1997, CHP earned over $1.9 billion in net revenues. Being a mission-driven health care delivery system poses unique challenges and opportunities in the health care industry in the United States. Nonetheless, CHP is currently blessed with some competent and visionary leaders who possess deep integrity and St. Mary's Health System is benefiting from that leadership talent.

Since joining the board at St. Mary's in 1991, I have gotten a unique opportunity to test my ideas about strategy and leadership as well as learn firsthand about this dynamic and complex industry. Because of this experience, I have been able to leverage my skills and understanding into several successful consulting engagements for other health care organizations, including a pharmaceutical firm, another health care delivery system, and a health care purchasing cooperative.

These experiences have revealed to me that much of the conventional wisdom of business schools does not apply to health care. For example, most health care organizations are not publicly traded and health care is fundamentally a service business. In contrast, most business theory and research is built around publicly-held, manufacturing-based corporations. As a result, conventional business thinking is often not applicable to many organizations in health care.

However, I am finding that cutting-edge ideas and practices in business are applicable. For example, as we move into an information-based economy, thinking about organizations in terms of core competencies (Prahalad & Hamel, 1990) with many opportunities for co-opetition (Brandenburger & Nalebuff, 1996) is useful and relevant to today's health care organization.

In particular, I am finding that the increasing emphasis on building value-creating strategic alliances between hospitals, physician groups, and insurance companies is the wave of the future (Kaluzny, Zuckerman, & Ricketts, 1995). The leaders who conceive and execute win-win-win partnerships between these three entities will be the ones who survive. Of course, this is easier said than done as health care has historically been a very fragmented industry and there are widely divergent interests and values and assumptions held within each of these three groups, not to mention between these groups. Nonetheless, it is critically important that the physician groups have trustworthy leadership to help with these changes. Consequently, I will rely on my five years of corporate experience, ten years of academic teaching and researching, and blend that with my eight years of experience with the health care industry to discuss physician leadership in the new millenium.

LEADERSHIP VERSUS MANAGEMENT

Many people use the terms leadership and management interchangeably, but this is a mistake because they are two fundamentally different sets of skills and abilities. In essence, management deals with the handling of resources within an existing organization while leadership deals with showing a new way of organizing and operating. According to one prominent leadership expert, managers create order; set impersonal goals, and have low emotional involvement with their work while leaders change the existing order of things, set very personal goals, and have a very high emotional involvement with their work (Zaleznick, 1977).

More recently, another prominent leadership expert argues that the manager's central function is to cope with complexity and their primary means of motivating others is organizational control systems and rewards. In contrast, the central function of leaders is to cope with change while attempting to inspire and empower the followers to enact the new order (Kotter, 1990).

The differences here are more than just semantics. If it is true that management is different from leadership (which I maintain is the correct perspective), then the selection, training, and educating of future leaders is somehow different from traditional management training (Heifetz & Laurie, 1997). Clearly, those in leadership roles also need to know management skills, but that is not enough because the requirements of the two jobs are fundamentally different.

My personal view is that preparing for a management position is largely technical in nature blended with adequate on-the-job experience while preparing for a leadership role is largely a matter of self awareness and character development blended with interpersonal skill (Badaracco, 1998; Judge, 1999). Both sets of skills are necessary for physician executives in the future, but they are not one in the same.

STRATEGIC LEADERSHIP

To be a leader, one must have followers. Consequently, leadership is fundamentally a relational phenomenon. Now there are all kinds of leadership positions—team leaders, department leaders, and organizational leaders come immediately to mind. However, as organizations become flatter and markets move more quickly, we are learning that leadership is not so much a position as it is a possibility for all people within an organization (Hughes, Ginnett, & Curphy, 1999). And progressive organizations are finding that it takes visionary strategic leadership at the apex of the organization to unleash the leadership potential within the rest of the organization (Finkelstein & Hambrick, 1996). Of course, not all people at the top of an organization are effective strategic leaders even though they occupy a pivotal position in the organization. However, strategic leadership is required of those who fill this role, especially physician executives who must strategically navigate a complex web of relationships (Blair & Fottler, 1998).

Strategic leadership may be conceived as a person or a group of persons, operating at the apex of the organization, who have found a way to balance their competencies and character in creative service of a larger vision of the future. The basic executive competencies involved are mainly the ability to exercise power and influence over the entire organization in a productive fashion. This is the traditional focus of most leadership assessment and training and is described in greater detail in Chapter 11. These competencies are critical abilities of all executive leaders and must not be neglected.

However, competency is not enough to be a strategic leader. One must also possess a developed character to be a strategic leader. Character is difficult to describe, impossible to teach, and confusing to explore. But like quality, everyone recognizes it when it is or is not present. Character is present when the person or persons are aware of their deeply held personal values and live according to those same values and principles. This is particularly important for physician leaders as they attempt to balance quality of care issues with financial constraints.

When senior people are viewed by their followers as competent and possessing character and integrity, then organizational trust grows and strategic change is possible. In the absence of either competence or character in those in leadership positions, self-interested behavior is often the norm within organizations and change usually is brought about only as desperate reactions to crises. Unfortunately, change brought about by crisis appears to be the norm in the health care industry today.

STRATEGIC LEADERSHIP COMPETENCIES

In addition to basic leadership competencies, strategic leaders need some higher order competencies to be effective. The first set of strategic competencies are in the area of strategic analysis. For example, Mike Stahl described SWOT analysis in Chapter 1. This ability to conceive and integrate the organization with its environment is paramount for strategic leaders.

Also, strategic leaders must know how to recognize the core competencies of their organization and invest in them heavily. In our increasingly interdependent economy, it is not possible nor is it feasible to be all things to all people. Organizations must figure out what they are best at and then find complementary organizations to collaborate with in order to create more and new customer value. By recognizing the one or two core competencies of the organization, its leaders know what to focus on internally and what to outsource. Strategic leaders often have to work with and sometimes change the corporate culture so an ability to do a cultural assessment is a critical skill (Goffee & Jones, 1996). Furthermore, strategic leaders must know how to develop and work with strategic scenarios in order to deal with the complexities and uncertainties of today's turbulent marketplace (Schwartz, 1991).

The second set of strategic leadership competencies is in the area of strategic change. Here, understanding of how the board of directors operates and basic ideas about corporate governance are essential. Knowing how to generate commitment to a course of action and balancing creativity with control are necessary. Also, an ability to develop and communicate a shared vision that inspires others is fundamental (Collins & Porras, 1994; Judge, 1999). Finally, knowing how to conceptualize and optimize the whole system, also known as systems thinking, is an increasingly important skill for strategic leaders, especially in health care. All of these skills are critical as physician practices grow in size, including those practices that affiliate with hospitals or health plans.

STRATEGIC LEADERSHIP CHARACTER

However, competency is not enough. The strategic leader must also have integrity of character to be effective. Leaders with integrity of character know their personal values and live consistently with them (Judge, 1999). They are less identified with their organizations and more identified with ideas and ideals. This identification allows them to shatter the status quo and seek creative new solutions to existing and future problems (Heifetz & Laurie, 1997).

To deal with all this change, the strategic leader must learn to become comfortable with ambiguity. As a result, another ingredient of integrity is the cultivation of higher than average tolerance for ambiguity. Further, since leadership is fundamentally a relational concept, one must be skilled in building and maintaining effective interpersonal relations. Hence, knowledge about one's interpersonal relations orientation is information that can assist in building integrity. Finally, awareness of the unique cognitive style of persons in an organization is essential to recognizing other styles that may be operating around oneself (Whetten & Cameron, 1995).

CONCLUSION

Leadership, particularly strategic leadership, is an important but difficult to teach phenomena that is critical to the effectiveness of every organization. Skill in leading others complements management skills, but these two sets of skills are not identical. Physicians have historically preferred to operate as independent entrepreneurs so the experience of management and leadership is often a new one to them. While much leadership is often learned through personal experience and trail and error, progressive leadership training and educational programs can facilitate this development process.

GLOSSARY

cognitive style. the way individuals gather and process information due to their personality preferences.

co-opetition. a new view of business where cooperation and competition are equally viable strategic alternatives to achieve business success based on the principles of game theory.

core competency. an integrated bundle of skills and technologies that contribute to an organization's competitive success.

corporate culture. the shared values within a firm that influence behaviors within that firm in powerful and often unconscious ways.

corporate governance. the entity legally responsible for the performance of the organization.

interpersonal relations orientation. the tendency to interact in certain ways with other people due to our inner attitudes toward inclusion, control, and affection.

organizational trust. the faith and confidence that members of an organization have in each other to act in ways that are competent, consistent, and benevolent.

personal values. deeply held beliefs that determine personal standards and desirable ends in life.

self-awareness. the depth by which we are conscious of our inner character.

shared vision. an image of the future that guides and inspires the entire organization.

strategic alliances. formal or informal partnerships between two or more organizations in order to achieve some mutually beneficial set of strategic objectives.

strategic change. a leadership ability to alter the organizational mindset and/or core competencies to make an organization more effective.

strategic leadership. the combination of character and skills of members of the top management team to help the organization achieve its financial and non-financial goals while developing future leaders in the organization.

strategic scenarios. tools for ordering one's perceptions about alternative future environments in which one's decisions might be played out.

systems thinking. a conceptual framework that makes overall patterns clearer and helps us to see how to change a system more effectively.

tolerance of ambiguity. the extent to which individuals are threatened by or have difficulty coping with situations that are uncertain, where change occurs rapidly or unpredictably, where information is unclear or inadequate, or where complexity exists.

REFERENCES

Badaracco, J. (1998). The discipline of building character. *Harvard Business Review, 98,* 115–124.

Blair, J., & Fottler, M. (1998). *Strategic leadership for medical groups.* San Francisco: Jossey–Bass.

Brandenburger, A., & Nalebuff, B. (1996). *Co-opetition.* New York: Doubleday.

Collins, J., & Porras, J. (1994). *Built to last.* New York: Harper Business.

Finkelstein, S., & Hambrick, D. (1996). *Strategic leadership.* St. Paul, MN: West Publishing.

Goffee, R., & Jones, G. (1996). What holds the modern company together? *Harvard Business Review, 74,* 133–148.

Hiefetz, R., & Laurie, D. (1997). The work of leadership. *Harvard Business Review, 75,* 124–134.

Hughes, R., Ginnett, R., & Curphy, G. (1999). *Leadership: Enhancing the lessons of experience* (3rd ed.). New York: Irwin/McGraw Hill.

Judge, W. (1999). *The leader's shadow: Exploring and developing executive character*. Beverly Hills, CA: Sage.

Kaluzny, A., Zuckerman, H., & Ricketts, T. (1995). *Partners for the dance: Forming strategic alliances in health care*. Ann Arbor, MI: Health Administration Press.

Kotter, J. (1990). What leaders really do. *Harvard Business Review, 90*, 103–111

Prahalad, C.K., & Hamel, G. (1990). The core competence of the corporation. *Harvard Business Review, May/June*, 79–91.

Schwartz, P. (1991). *The art of the long view*. New York: Doubleday Currency.

Zaleznick, A. (1977). Managers and leaders: Are they different? *Harvard Business Review, 55*, 67–78.

Whetten, D., & Cameron, K. (1995). *Developing management skills* (3rd ed). New York: HarperCollins Publishers.

CHAPTER 11

Transitioning Leadership Styles: Physicians Preparing for Health Care Leadership

*Kate P. Atchley, Laura A. Gniatczyk,
Robert T. Ladd and Todd W. Little**

TABLE OF CONTENTS

---

*Note: All authors contributed equally to the preparation of this chapter and are therefore listed in alphabetical order.

EXECUTIVE SUMMARY

The role of physicians is shifting from that of caregivers to that of business leaders in the dynamic health care industry. This chapter elaborates on the need for physicians to focus on improving their management and leadership skills. In order for these changes in leadership style to occur, physicians must familiarize themselves with their current skill levels and identify developmental needs. The authors propose means for accomplishing these goals. In addition, both formal and informal assessment techniques are enumerated, as well as the process for pursuing a personal development plan.

INTRODUCTION

It would be folly to contend that a physician enrolls in a Masters of Business Administration program for the purpose of improving her or his skills as a physician. While an increased understanding of the business world may afford the physician increased flexibility within the practice of medicine, this benefit is unquestionably minimal with respect to the cost of the degree in terms of both time and money. Rather, the most logical reason for a physician enrolling in a MBA program is to expand her or his role beyond that of professional caregiver and amateur manager to that of a leader, a leader in the multifaceted, continuously evolving, bureaucratic and often confusing field which is modern health care.

A physician desiring a leadership role within health care should anticipate numerous difficulties and changes. Improving the various systems which makeup modern health care requires more than knowledge; it requires the ability to recognize issues, formulate change strategies, utilize human resources, and influence decisions. Medical schools, however, do nothing to prepare physicians to take this leadership role. Rather, physicians are taught to do their best within the system, not to change the system (Berwick & Nolan, 1998). Physicians approaching the leadership role must therefore focus on changing their view of the system and their interpersonal style. Among other things, this changed focus requires adapting to new environments and dealing effectively with non-physicians.

Many physicians and management consultants have attempted to define the leadership role. Focusing on medicine, Bogdewic, Baxley, and Jamison (1997) consolidated numerous theorists' formulations into five leadership competencies. In general, their competencies incorporate interpersonal skills with system management principles, including: (1) "to develop a shared vision and direct attention to shared goals"; (2) "to communicate a sense of purpose or meaning in long-range vision and department goals"; (3) "to foster collaboration and cooperation"; (4) "to empower and honor others, value diverse perspectives and talent"; and (5) "to establish trust through behavior that is consistent with values and beliefs (p. 263)." Each of these competencies require effecting some strategic or organization-wide goal through the use of some set of unspecified but highly individualized skills. Leadership, therefore, is concerned first with what is accomplished, but also incorporates numerous means, most interpersonally based, in accomplishing this goal.

If a physician enters a MBA program out of a desire to move into a leadership role, then the responsive program should address each physician's development into a leader. Certainly the course content should aid the physician in understanding the systems involved in health care organizations. Finance and accounting systems, operational management, and continuous improvement systems are all important in establishing an understanding and respect for systems outside those typically associated with a physician practicing medicine. Hopefully, this understanding will in turn foster a better strategic perspective, better relationships within the system, and a continuous improvement of health care systems. Nevertheless, specific attention to the means through which a physician leader asserts leadership within an organization is also appropriate. Bogdewic et al. (1997) suggest that this development must begin with introspection, and should then proceed through individual initiatives targeted at optimizing the physician leader's leadership skill and style.

Individualization with regard to leadership development is necessary due to the wide variety of interpersonal skills and styles possessed by physicians. Interestingly, a retrospective assessment of individuals entering Executive MBA (EMBA) programs at the University of Tennessee suggest that physicians are not unlike most other individuals entering an EMBA program. Like many professionals who have had successful careers, physicians pursuing such a program are often solid problem solvers with a wide variety of interpersonal styles. In fact, when the self-reported interpersonal styles of physicians and non-physicians entering the EMBA programs were compared, no significant group differences were noted. In general, both groups possessed strong cognitive abilities but highly varied personalities. No general description of the physician or executive leader could be developed. Accordingly, no general model for leadership development was deemed appropriate. Physician EMBA students (and other EMBA students) range from moderately introverted individuals who are adaptive and efficient, to strongly extroverted individuals who are dominant and forceful. Their values are also highly individualized. Some physicians are flexible and accepting of others' ideas, while others are dogmatic and intolerant of differences and change. Some achieve through conformity, while others seek and excel in highly independent situations. Many are highly sociable, but some eschew social situations. All in all, there is no one model for a person seeking an EMBA degree or a leadership role in health care or other organizations.

Despite the wide variety of individual differences observed, there are a number of common themes associated with health care leadership roles. First, leadership requires building vision or purpose. This necessitates looking outside medicine for answers. Physicians should understand how the market system operates and how other professions have managed change. In addition, physician leaders must be able to recognize unproductive processes within the present health care system. All of these requirements demand interactions with other disciplines and professions and an understanding of health care systems from multiple perspectives (Zismer, Fansler, & Porter, 1991). Further, leadership mandates understanding processes and how individuals contribute to those processes. Physician leaders should facilitate rather than provide solutions. That is, leaders must enable others to solve problems rather than solving the problems themselves (Reinertsen, 1998). Thus, they employ interpersonal influence to promote the development of others. Finally, leadership requires the confidence and courage to act. This necessitates practice, feedback, and more practice in disciplines and functions outside the traditional role of caregiver.

In summary, the task of developing a physician leader requires assessment of knowledge and skills, understanding systems outside of medicine, and the development of interpersonal skills to facilitate leadership. In order to prepare for a new leadership/managerial position, it is essential that the physician allocate some time for self-assessment. While it is often difficult to be honest regarding personal strengths and weaknesses, some amount of introspection is required prior to skill development. In general, there are several ways to go about skill assessment: formal means, informal means, or some combination of both.

SKILL ASSESSMENT

Formal Assessment

Formal assessments typically involve receiving assistance from a professional person or service that has experience with providing such information. The physician leader should expect this formal approach to involve a variety of simulated assessments, evaluations of current performance, and written tests (including personality inventories and cognitive assessments). This chapter examines some of the alternatives available through a formal assessment process. Specifically, performance feedback obtained via a 360-degree feedback instrument, skill assessments generated from a developmental assessment center, and additional assessment tools will be discussed.

360-Degree Feedback Instruments

A 360-degree feedback system is a performance appraisal method which utilizes information obtained from multiple, diverse sources to provide comprehensive feedback to individuals. The popularity of 360-degree feedback systems has greatly increased in the past ten years. In fact, recent surveys indicate that approximately 15% of organizations in the United States utilize some type of 360-degree feedback program (Yammarino & Atwater, 1997). These systems are considered to provide more extensive feedback than traditional performance ratings made only by supervisors.

Physician leaders regularly interact with people at many different levels within an organization (e.g., nurses, other doctors, board of directors, office staff). A 360-degree feedback instrument is unique in that it incorporates feedback from multiple raters at each of these levels. In addition to self ratings, a 360-degree feedback typically includes ratings by direct supervisors, peers, direct reports, and even customers (i.e., patients). External customers are sometimes excluded because the behaviors they observe are so different from those seen by the other raters (Bracken, 1994). The varying perspectives offered by the raters combine to give the ratee a more global view of his or her strengths and weaknesses. The logic underlying this process should be rather intuitive—who better to assess work-related skills than the people the physician leader works with on a daily basis (Kiechel, 1989)?

The implementation of a 360-degree feedback appraisal system is relatively straightforward. The primary criterion for choosing a rater is simply that they have had ample opportunity to observe job-relevant behaviors (Bracken, 1994). The actual appraisal instrument should be tailored to the respective organization and target specific behaviors rather than traits. In other words, it should focus on what the physician leader actually does or does not do (e.g., provides feedback to subordinates; conveys his or her thoughts clearly when speaking) rather than general personality traits (e.g., domineering, sociable; Bracken, 1994). Questionnaire items typically begin with an active verb followed by a phrase that specifies the target behavior. For example, "At work [the physician] treats each employee as an individual and shows that he or she is truly concerned about them." These items are rated on a multi-point scale (e.g., strongly agree to strongly disagree). In addition to these ratings, raters are sometimes given the opportunity to answer open-ended questions about the ratee in order to provide detailed feedback not specifically addressed in the questionnaire. If answered thoughtfully, these unstructured responses to the open-ended questions can be a valuable contribution to the complete feedback picture. It is extremely important to maintain the anonymity of the rater throughout the feedback process; otherwise, raters may not feel comfortable providing honest feedback. This is usually accomplished by enlisting an external person or organization to compile the ratings and generate reports for the ratees. The report enables the physician to identify both strengths and areas for improvement as identified by others. This information can then be used to establish developmental goals.

The use of 360-degree feedback instruments as both developmental tools and as part of formal appraisal systems has increased dramatically in recent years. The fact that people are often surprised by how others perceive their strengths and weaknesses makes the feedback particularly valuable. Though rating sources do not always agree (e.g., peer ratings may be in sharp contrast to employee ratings), this reinforces the fact that behaviors may be differentially observed by different groups of coworkers in the same work setting. The primary goal of 360-degree feedback is for the ratee to see him or herself through the "eyes" of his or her coworkers. However, the physician leader undergoing this process should not attempt to anticipate the results that he or she will receive. For example, while most people rate themselves high with respect to people skills, coworkers often don't agree (Kiechel, 1989). Similarly, only about one-third of self-assessments actually match those provided by coworkers (O'Reilly, 1994), and of the remaining two-thirds, half of the self-assessments are inflated when compared to coworkers (O'Reilly, 1994). These discrepancies only accentuate the benefits of 360-degree feedback.

Assessment Centers

Assessment centers are a system, rather than a place, in which situational exercises are used to evaluate the specific behavior of the participant(s) (Thornton, 1992). Participation in an assessment center typically takes anywhere from half a day to multiple days and requires participants to interact in both one-on-one and group situations. Additionally, most assessment centers also require participants to complete a number of written exercises that do not require interaction with others, but instead require individuals to respond in a written format to a number of issues or make decisions based upon material presented to them. Assessment centers have commonly been used to make selection decisions and/or provide developmental feedback. While an accurate estimate on the total usage of assessment centers is not available, anecdotal information suggests that they are now widely used for everything from manufacturing, police, fire, and management hiring to career development programs.

Assessment centers focus on assessing certain behavioral tendencies or dimension-relevant behaviors exhibited by participants. Dimensions are defined as "clusters of behaviors that are specific, observable and verifiable, and that can be reliably and logically classified together" (Thornton & Byham, 1982, p. 117). Dimensions that are typically evaluated include analysis, judgment, planning and organizing, delegation, written and oral communication, and leadership. In order to make accurate assessments of the relevant dimensions, assessment center participants complete multiple exercises. In most cases, a dimension is evaluated in at least two exercises, so that participants' behavior can be observed in a variety of situations. Furthermore, information obtained through an assessment center is typically combined with results on written tests such as cognitive ability or personality instruments. These types of instruments will be discussed later in this chapter.

Exercises that are typically included in an assessment center are: simulated one-on-one interactions, leaderless group discussions, case analysis exercises, and in-basket exercises (Thornton, 1992; Thornton & Byham, 1982). Simulated interactions are usually relatively short exercises in which the participant interacts with an assessment center staff member acting in the capacity of a role player. These exercises are particularly effective at elucidating "oral communication skill, empathy and tact, and problem-solving ability with people" (Thornton, 1992, p. 70). Similarly, leaderless group discussions (LGD) are also effective at eliciting oral communication and problem-solving ability, as well as leadership, orientation toward team work, and willingness to initiate action. In a LGD, it is typical for 3 or more assessment center participants to be provided a task which requires a decision in a certain period of time (typically 45 minutes to 1 hour). This exercise is called an LGD because none of the group members have been assigned the role of leader and therefore someone must either adopt the role or all members must share the role of leader in order to achieve the goal. During both the simulated one-on-one interaction and the LGD, participants are observed by trained assessment center staff members who are responsible for recording behavior during the exercises and then evaluating these behaviors once the exercise is completed.

While the simulated one-on-one interaction and the LGD are interpersonal exercises, the case analysis exercise and the in-basket are written tasks that are completed by the participant and evaluated by the assessment center staff upon completion of the exercise. The case analysis exercise presents the participant with information on a company and allows for the observation of a participant's ability to "sift through data, recognize and document organizational problems, generate alternate solutions, and formulate defensible solutions" (Thornton & Byham, 1982, p. 191). Similarly, in the in-basket exercise, participants are provided a variety of documents which include memoranda, letters, chart/graphs, phone messages, a calendar, and irrelevant information. These materials are meant to reflect the contents of an individual's In-Box at work. Assessment center participants are required to respond to the various stimulus materials in writing. Typical dimensions assessed via the in-basket exercise include planning and organizing, initiative, delegation, and judgment.

It is important to note that there is no one standard compilation of exercises but rather the exercises selected should reflect the skills necessary for the target position. In other words, individuals participating in a developmental assessment center should complete exercises which emphasize the skills needed in the desired position. For example, physician leaders aspiring to management or leadership positions should focus on skills like decision making, planning and organizing, and customer orientation.

Upon completion of the assessment center, participants should be provided with detailed feedback that reviews the individual's relative strengths and weaknesses by dimension. Specific details should be provided so that the participants can use the feedback to make adjustments to their current style. In addition to reviewing written feedback, all participants in a developmental assessment center should have the opportunity to discuss their results with an individual trained in the assessment center methodology. More information about this interaction will be discussed in the coaching section.

Additional Assessment Tools

To supplement the feedback that can be generated using the 360-degree feedback process and/or assessment centers, it is possible that the feedback seeker will be asked to complete cognitive ability instruments (e.g., *Watson-Glaser Critical Thinking Appraisal,* 1980; *Wechsler Adult Intelligence Scale*, Wechsler, 1981; *Wonderlic Basic Skills Test*, Long, Artese, & Clonts, 1995) and/or personality instruments (e.g., *California Psychological Inventory*, Gough, 1996; *Hogan Personality Inventory*; Hogan, 1986; *Sixteen Personality Factor Questionaire*, Cattell & Stice, 1957). These types of measures are typically paper and pencil instruments that are administered, scored, and interpreted by trained professionals, and the results of these instruments can provide useful information to augment a feedback report. For example, if an individual completes a personality instrument and is found to be extremely introverted, this data can be helpful in explaining his or her reticence during a leaderless group discussion. The physician leader is encouraged to complete these types of instruments because, ultimately, the resulting data will aid in the interpretation of his or her behaviors exhibited during the assessment center or identified in the 360-degree feedback process.

Informal Assessment

In addition to the multitude of formal assessment methods, there are numerous informal assessment tools available to the proactive physician leader. These may include anything from internal services offered by employers (e.g., career planning, continuing education programs) to self-evaluation instruments published in books. In addition, self-evaluation tools are available via the Internet and popular press books found at a local library or bookstore. Although these types of tools lack the depth of formal methods discussed earlier in this chapter, they are usually relatively inexpensive, easy to use, and are generally suitable for increasing self–awareness.

Informal assessments consist of appraisal instruments that physician leaders can usually administer and/or interpret themselves. They typically involve some level of personal introspection through which physicians honestly appraise their own skill sets. One alternative available to most physicians is to simply use the feedback received as part of an organization's formal performance appraisal as a springboard for beginning a self-directed development process. The physician leader's superiors are also an excellent source of information; when approached, superiors are generally quite willing to assist employees in identifying developmental areas. Additionally, close confidants and associates are good people to ask for constructive feedback. Due to their familiarity with the physician leader, their feedback is often particularly salient. This recommendation obviously assumes a certain level of trust in the relationship, thus allowing the feedback giver to feel entirely comfortable providing honest responses without fear of reprisal. In the absence of a formal skill assessment process, it is highly recommended that several informal assessment tools are utilized by the physician leader in order to obtain a more complete self-diagnosis.

SKILL DEVELOPMENT

Once formal or informal skill assessments have been used to identify areas for development, there are a variety of skill development options available to the physician leader. These include self-improvement seminars, continuing education courses, career planning workshops, one-on-one coaching, and implementing a personal development plan. This portion of the chapter focuses on one-on-one coaching and personal development planning, two of the most comprehensive approaches to enhancing the physician leader's skills.

One-on-One Coaching

As a part of the formal assessment process, the physician leader may be paired with a facilitator, or coach, who is trained in executive development techniques. Coaching is increasing in popularity as a developmental tool for physician leaders and executives. The coaching process can be defined as a sequence of one-on-one meetings between a facilitator and a physician leader with the purpose of improving the physician leader's job performance. Though the original intent of coaching was to work with executives who demonstrated potential but needed to improve their skills, coaching is becoming quite common as a way for high-potential leaders to further hone their skills (Judge & Cowell, 1997). Due to the highly individualized nature of the coaching process, it makes sense that coaching is becoming viewed as a time-effective development process to help a physician leader fully realize his or her potential.

The individual serving as a coach may take on many different roles in the course of the relationship, including trainer, motivator, sounding board, and devil's advocate (Judge & Cowell, 1997). While the coach identifies and helps to address a physician leader's weaknesses, it is critical to note that the coach's role should not be that of a psychotherapist or personal counselor. Effective coaches are individuals that have a background in psychological theory and adult learning theory, as well as a broad understanding of the many aspects of business and government (e.g., finance, production, marketing, customer relations, political savvyness, etc.). A working knowledge of a multitude of industries, business trends, and current affairs are also components of being an effective coach (Levinson, 1996).

Typical coaching methods include the following (Kilburg, 1996):

- Skill assessment (e.g., personality inventories, reasoning tests, 360-degree surveys, etc.)
- Feedback sessions
- Interviewing peers and employees about the physician leader's skills
- Assignment of readings
- Role playing
- Feedback on written documents
- Introducing the physician leader to needed resources (e.g., experts in a specific field of study, textbooks, etc.)
- Suggesting educational workshops that address specific weaknesses
- Crisis interventions
- Organizational assessment

A coach's job is typically a 5-step process: First, the coach assesses the physician leader's behavioral skill set using some of the previously discussed methodologies (e.g., 360-degree survey, assessment center, personality inventories, cognitive ability tests). Second, the coach provides extensive feedback to the physician leader on the effectiveness of his or her skills. The coach utilizes graphical representations of the collected data, content analysis of interviews, and test scores to present feedback to the physician leader. Third, the coach aids the physician leader in articulating a desired state of performance and identifying the skill gaps that are keeping the physician leader from attaining that level of performance. Fourth, the coach then aids the physician leader in outlining a plan of action to enhance skill acquisition. Lastly, the coach follows up with the physician leader to assess progress in skill development. An implicit assumption in all five steps is that the physician leader is an *active* participant in the process. By combining a coach's skills and objective observations with a physician leader's expertise and understanding of his or her organization, a physician leader can realize faster results (Witherspoon & White, 1996).

Creating a Development Plan

A development plan is a formalized set of goals and actions to be taken in pursuit of those goals for the purpose of increasing skills, knowledge, or experience. An underlying assumption of the creation of a development plan is that the most effective way to help physician leaders expand their skills is to encourage their active involvement in establishing goals for their own development and career growth (Wexley & Latham, 1991). Nothing is an adequate substitute for the physician leader's self-awareness of developmental needs and motivation to improve his or her personal management or leadership style.

The first step a physician leader should take in creating a meaningful development plan is the examination of his or her strengths and weaknesses. For each source of feedback data available, the physician leader should list those skills assessed as strengths, competencies, or weaknesses. For example, if the physician leader has 360-degree survey results, a separate list of perceived skills and areas for improvement should be made for each data source (e.g., one list for peers, one list for subordinates, one list for self, etc.). Another example is that of an assessment center feedback report: based on the behavioral incidents present in the report, a listing of those behaviors performed effectively and ineffectively by the physician leader should be made.

After all the data has been examined, it is important that the physician leader take time to integrate the information across the different sources of data. Are there trends in the data? Are certain strengths or weaknesses consistently mentioned across the different sources in the physician leader's feedback? It is this triangulation of data that serves to validate the need for augmentation of a particular skill. For example, the physician leader may have performed poorly in the assessment center on the delegation dimension, and subordinates' perception of his or her delegation skills were reported as weak in the 360-degree survey results. These two indications, combined with the physician leader's self-awareness of discomfort with delegation (e.g., a belief that it is easier to perform a task by one's self than teach someone else how to do it; an extremely full plate of tasks that never seems to decrease), should indicate to the physician leader that delegation is a key skill that should be targeted for improvement.

Once deficiencies are identified, the physician leader then begins articulating goals and developing a plan of action to improve these skills. A goal is defined as "anything an individual is consciously trying to achieve" (Wexley & Latham, 1991, p. 90). Goals are very important because without them, individuals have virtually no basis for evaluating their progress or measuring their abilities. While it is advisable to target multiple skills for improvement, the physician leader should prioritize these goals in order to allocate an appropriate amount of time to each goal. Recognize that skill development is a time consuming task; the time and effort required to effect change in one's skill level should not be underestimated.

Goal setting is an established technique for self-improvement (Locke & Latham, 1984). Research conducted on goal setting has several implications for motivating physician leaders. First, an individual must have the conviction that he or she can reach the goal; this is called a person's self-efficacy (Bandura, 1986). Second, specific goals result in higher levels of performance than ambiguous goals, and moderately difficult goals result in higher levels of performance than easy goals. Third, a large goal should be broken down into subgoals, or distinct, feasible steps that the physician leader can achieve in a timely manner. Achievement of subgoals provides a feeling of accomplishment, sustains a individual's motivation level and enhances his or her self-efficacy.

It is also important that specific activities are listed that can be pursued to help develop the identified skill and that can be tracked to assess progress in reaching the goal. See Exhibit 11–1 for an example of a plan outlined to improve oral presentation skills.

In a completely self-directed development process, the physician leader is responsible for monitoring his or her own progress toward goal attain-

Exhibit 11–1 An Example of a Developmental Goal and Action Plan

<u>**Goal:**</u>	**Become more comfortable delivering oral presentations.**
<u>**Plan:**</u>	
(A)	I will deliver at least two presentations during the next quarter.
(B)	I will solicit feedback from my peers attending the presentations using a checklist of effective behaviors.
(C)	I will prepare outlines defining the purpose of my presentation to prevent rambling.
(D)	I will read a popular press book about effective presentations.
(E)	I will volunteer as a lay liturgist at my church once per month and use that opportunity to focus on speaking with inflection and maintaining eye contact.

ment. However, some physician leaders may find it useful to enlist the counsel of a one-on-one coach for expert guidance and to serve as an external accountability mechanism.

Whether the physician leader decides to hire a coach or outline a self-directed development program, it is very important that the physician leader develops a method for tracking his or her progress. This can look like a weekly checklist of activities, journal or diary entries, or notes in a planner. Periodically reexamining goals and activities also enhances the development plan. As certain goals are reached, new goals can be established. In addition, reviewing which activities are effective or ineffective for skill development allows the physician leader the opportunity to substitute more feasible plans of action.

It is important to note that the aforementioned formal and informal assessment and development methods are not an exhaustive list of options, nor are the formal and informal methods mutually exclusive. The physician leader is encouraged to employ any combination of methods that suits his or her individualized needs. True leadership development is a constant in the physician leader's life, preparing him or her for whatever changes the health care industry may bring in the future.

Regardless of the methods utilized, it is important that physician leaders remember that skill assessment and development are just the first two steps in what will become, ideally, a life-long learning process. Once physician leaders are comfortable with the process of self evaluation, they can begin to incorporate this into their daily routine. Physician leaders should understand the importance of seeking continuous feedback on their skills, refinement of goals based on this feedback, and the establishment of new goals to meet the needs of the dynamic health care environment.

GLOSSARY

assessment center. an evaluative procedure which utilizes multiple exercises to appraise a physician leader's competency in relevant skill/ability areas.

case analysis exercise. a method frequently used in an assessment center to assess physician leaders' abilities to comprehend and integrate data presented to them.

coaching. a one-on-one relationship between a physician leader and a professional facilitator with the objective of improving job performance.

cognitive ability instrument. a formal test administered to examine an individual's mental ability.

360-degree feedback. a performance appraisal method in which coworkers rate the physician leader on various work-related behaviors.

development plan. a formalized set of goals and actions to be taken in pursuit of those goals for the purpose of increasing skills, knowledge, or experience.

dimension. a group of specific, observable behaviors that can be logically combined and labeled under one heading.

formal assessment. a process in which a physician leader receives assistance from a professional person or organization that has experience with providing skill assessment and development feedback.

goal setting. an established technique for self-improvement that involves outlining specific, difficult goals and distinct steps for achieving each goal.

in-basket exercise. a method frequently used in an assessment center that tests the physician leader's ability to prioritize and resolve a multitude of business-related issues.

informal assessment. consists of self-directed activities, such as introspection, talking with confidants, completing self-assessment instruments, etc., that results in useful information concerning the physician leader's personal skill development needs.

leaderless group discussion. a method frequently used in an assessment center that involves the interaction of small groups of individuals who are charged with the task of solving a problem. In addition, no formal roles are assigned to any group members, necessitating the use of interpersonal skills in a group setting.

personality instrument. an inventory designed to measure the unique characteristics which define an individual and to identify his or her tendencies in interacting with people, things, and situations.

ratee. the physician leader who is the target of the performance appraisal questionnaire (e.g., 360-degree feedback instruments).

rater. the individual(s) that provide(s) the ratings for the target individual.

role playing. a technique where a physician leader is asked to place him—or herself in an imaginary situation for the purpose of gaining insight and practice with interpersonal skills.

simulated one-on-one interaction(s). a method frequently used in an assessment center to assess a physician leader's ability to work individually and face-to-face with co-workers in a variety of business-related situations.

sub-goals. distinct, feasible steps that the physician leader can achieve in a timely manner in pursuit of a larger goal.

REFERENCES

Bandura, A. (1986). *Social foundations of thought and action*. Englewood Cliffs, NJ: Prentice Hall.

Berwick, D.M., & Nolan, T.W. (1998). Physicians as leaders in improving health care: A new series in annals of internal medicine. *Annals of Internal Medicine, 128,* 289–292.

Bogdewic, S.P., Baxley, E.G., & Jamison, P.K. (1997). Leadership and organizational skills in academic medicine. *Family Medicine, 29,* 262–265.

Bracken, D.W. (1994, September). Straight talk about multirater feedback. *Training & Development,* 44–51.

Cattell, R.B., & Stice, G.F. (1957). *Handbook for the sixteen personality factor questionnaire.* Champaign, IL: Institute of Personality and Ability Testing.

Gough, H.G. (1996). *CPI Manual* (3rd ed.). Palto Alto, CA: Consulting Psychologists Press, Inc.

Hogan, R. (1986). *Manual for the Hogan personality inventory.* Minneapolis, MN: National Computer Systems.

Judge, W.Q., & Cowell, J. (1997). The brave new world of executive coaching. *Business Horizons, 40,* 71–77.

Kiechel, W. (1989, June 19). When subordinates evaluate the boss. *Fortune*, 201–202.

Kilburg, R.R. (1996). Toward a conceptual understanding and definition of executive coaching. *Consulting Psychology Journal: Practice and Research, 48,* 134–144.

Levinson, H. (1996). Executive coaching. *Consulting Psychology Journal: Practice and Research, 48,* 115–123.

Locke, E.A., & Latham, G.P. (1984). *A theory of goal setting and task performance.* Englewood Cliffs, NJ: Prentice Hall.

Long, E.R., Artese, V.S., & Clonts, W.L. (1995). *Wonderlic Basic Skills Test.* Libertyville, IL: Wonderlic Personnel Test, Inc.

O'Reilly, B. (1994, October 17). 360 feedback can change your life. *Fortune,* 93–100.

Reinertsen, J.L. (1998). Physicians as leaders in the improvement of health care systems. *Annals of Internal Medicine, 128,* 833–838.

Thornton, G.C. (1992). *Assessment centers in human resource management.* Reading, MA: Addison Wesley Publishing Co.

Thornton, G.C., & Byham, W.C. (1982). *Assessment centers and managerial performance.* San Diego, CA: Academic Press.

Watson, G., & Glaser, E.M. (1980). *Watson-Glaser Critical Thinking Appraisal Manual.* New York: The Psychological Corporation.

Wechsler, D. (1981). *Manual for the Wechsler Adult Intelligence Scale—Revised.* New York: The Psychological Corporation.

Wexley, K.N., & Latham, G.P. (1991). *Developing and training human resources in organizations.* New York: HarperCollins Publishers.

Witherspoon, R., & White, R.P. (1996). Executive coaching: A continuum of roles. *Consulting Psychology Journal: Practice and Research, 48,* 124–133.

Yammarino, F.J., & Atwater, L.E. (1997). Do managers see themselves as others see them? Implications of self-other rating agreement for human resources management. *Organizational Dynamics, 25,* 35–44.

Zismer, D.K., Fransler, D.D., & Porter, S. (1991). The physician as organizational leader. *Minnesota Medicine, 74,* 37–38.

CHAPTER 12

Business Law and Business Ethics for Physician Leaders

Peter J. Dean and Cheryl S. Massingale

TABLE OF CONTENTS

EXECUTIVE SUMMARY

Physician leaders, who trained for many years to provide the best available patient care, find themselves in a new arena in the late 1990s. Physicians can no longer focus entirely on the provision of health care services to patients. In a pre-managed care environment, physicians relied on the standards of the latest medical research, some law, and well–documented medical ethics to guide them in their practice of medicine. Now, physicians must negotiate an unfamiliar minefield of business decisions, contract negotiations, strategic planning issues, and statutory and regulatory hurdles. Physicians must also understand and appreciate that medical ethics and business ethics are the same, but different. Today, the knowledge of business law and business ethics is critical for the practice of medicine and an essential ingredient in executive MBA programs. This chapter addresses some of the issues important to physician leaders facing myriad business decisions and confounded by legal and ethical headaches in today's health care environment.

LEGAL ISSUES IN THE BUSINESS OF HEALTH CARE

Health care has become an increasingly regulated field, and the focus on health care crime and wrongdoing is unprecedented. Although the legal issues facing physicians are numerous, a few issues are particularly problematic for providers in the managed care arena. Three areas that have proven to be especially difficult include: (1) contracting in the managed care environment, (2) antitrust and price fixing issues for providers, and (3) fraud and abuse. These topics are relevant to all physicians practicing in a managed care environment and all physician leaders managing in that environment due to increased legal exposure and more aggressive enforcement efforts.

Contracting in a Managed Care Environment

Prior to the emergence of managed care, physicians provided care and hospitals provided the place for much of that care. Insurers, private and governmental, provided most of the payment for care. There were relatively few incidents requiring physicians to enter into complex contracts within their profession beyond the lease or purchase of office space and partnership agreements among members of a group practice. Physicians independently controlled treatment and admission decisions and the scope of their practices was a function of their individual ability to attract and retain patients. Physicians generally enjoyed good working relationships with other physicians and health care professionals. Any competition within the profession was more or less friendly. Roles were clearly defined and the credo seemed to be "more is better." This position was both legally and ethically sound given the belief that more tests led to better diagnoses, and longer hospital stays ensured faster and more complete recoveries. During this time medical research flourished, producing better drugs, better tools, and more sophisticated machines and techniques. While enabling better care, these advancements also contributed to the rising cost of health care. The payers began to look for ways to control costs. One strategy to deal with the rising costs was the expansion of the market-driven force of managed care. Managed care, as it has evolved, might more correctly be called "managed cost." Managed care plans attempt to control costs in part by rationing care to patients. Under managed care, physicians, like many other suppliers of health care services, are called providers. Managed care plans negotiate with providers to procure services at fees that are substantially less than their ordinary fees. In return, providers are assured a broad patient base. But these arrangements often require that providers relinquish a great deal of their autonomy in providing care. Decisions regarding treatment protocols, referrals, hospital admissions, and lengths of stays are now subject to review and approval by health care plan administrators. Even choices of prescription drugs may be determined by the terms of the health care plan.

In an effort to increase their marketability and negotiating power vis-a-vis health plans, providers align in single or multi-specialty groups (horizontal integration) or with other provider groups such as hospitals, pharmaceutical companies, or insurance groups (vertical integration). As physicians jockey to form networks with payers and other providers, the contracting process becomes very complex. Issues such as pricing of services, levels of risk, methods of reimbursement, and how to get out of the contract if the arrangement doesn't work out are but a few of the perplexing contract terms that must be negotiated. While an in-depth discussion of these contracts is beyond the scope of this chapter, some potential missteps for physician leaders are discussed below.

Antitrust and Price Fixing

As providers combine to form new groups and gain bargaining strength, antitrust issues loom as a real threat for the unwary provider. The idea that antitrust issues are only related to monolithic companies and that price fixing is only connected to criminals trying to squeeze out competitors is long since passe. The purpose of anti-competitive laws, under the broad title of antitrust, is to ensure free competition in the marketplace. In a market economy, competition is considered to be the most appropriate way to increase quality and reduce prices. Both federal and state laws govern antitrust issues, with state laws varying somewhat among the differing states. Federal law, however, provides clear prohibitions to anti-competitive activities and imposes severe penalties for violations.

Government authorities analyze suspected antitrust violations using either *per se* or rule of reason analysis. Violations deemed to be *per se* violations are indefensible, regardless of good intent or positive market effects. Rule of reason analysis requires inquiry into the arrangement to determine whether it promotes or interferes with competition (Cohen, 1997). In the health care context, an investigated provider would have the opportunity to justify a given arrangement or action under the rule of reason, but not if the action is determined to be a *per se* violation.

The antitrust issues most relevant in health care are monopolies, anti-competitive mergers, illegal boycotts, market allocation, and price fixing. A monopoly occurs when a group possesses the ability to control prices or to exclude competitors. Where a provider group gains too large a share of the relevant market, or gains monopoly power, it stifles competition and violates antitrust law. Section 2 of the Sherman Act (1890) prohibits all attempts or conspiracies to monopolize. The test generally used to determine the degree of power is market share. A market share greater than 75% generally indicates market power, while less than 50% market share suggests a lack of market power (Mann & Roberts, 1997). In health care, these threshold percentages are likely to be somewhat smaller. Unlike other forms of anti-competitive behavior, monopoly violations can occur through the acts of a single group and do not require agreements or activities among competitors. In the health care context, violations can occur where groups obtain too large a share of the relevant market, and it can be shown that they have the ability to affect prices or competition and that they have willfully acquired or maintained that power.

Mergers are one means of acquiring market share, and federal enforcers are paying close attention to group practice mergers that may threaten competition (Klein, 1998). The Federal law that governs mergers is Section 7 of the Clayton Act. This section prohibits mergers, joint ventures, consolidations, and acquisitions of stock or assets where the effect may be to substantially lessen competition or create a monopoly. Merger enforcement in health care appears to be focused on very large single or multi-specialty groups because these mega-groups tend to be a draw to health plans and employers, but discourage new entries to the market, thus limiting competitors (Klein, 1998). Mergers of competitors in rural or narrowly defined markets which create a very large market share may be more suspect than mergers that occur in large markets with many competitors.

Antitrust violations occur not only when significant market shares are involved but also with any activity that interferes with free competition. Section I of the Sherman Act prohibits contracts, combinations, and conspiracies that create a restraint of trade. Subsequent court decisions have construed the act to prohibit only *unreasonable* restraints of trade (Chicago Board of Trade v. United States, 1918). Section 1 does not apply to unilateral acts, but requires agreements or combinations. Boycotts are one kind of restraint of trade that present a significant pitfall for physicians. As private or government plans apply more and more cost-cutting pressure on providers, a common temptation for providers is to agree among themselves to refuse to do business with the offending plan under the proposed terms. If such an agreement is between competitors, the activity constitutes an illegal boycott which may initiate severe penalties on the unsuspecting physicians. Illegal boycotts occur when two or more groups agree not to deal with a third party. Therefore, a single provider group can decide not to do business with another person, business, or plan, and that would not violate antitrust laws. But if competitors conspire or agree to refuse to do business with a third party, it may constitute an illegal boycott in violation of Section 1 of the Sherman Act. The same rationale applies with market allocation among competitors. If providers agree to divide the market, either geographically or by services offered, it will constitute a *per se* violation of the Sherman Act. This activity interferes with competition and threatens to raise prices to consumers.

The most serious example of a *per se* violation of the Sherman Act is price fixing. Agreements among competitors with the intent or effect of affecting prices constitutes illegal price fixing. Whether the agreement is meant to establish maximum prices or minimum prices at which a service will be offered or it was intended to improve the quantity of the service offered, it is prohibited under the Sherman Act. In a managed care environment, any agreement among providers to establish the price at which services would be offered to a health care plan or an agreement among plans to establish maximum prices to be paid for given services would be price fixing. Price-fixing violations among competing providers are seldom as blatant as overt agreements on how much each will charge for a given procedure or service, but they present a hidden trap when pricing information is shared as provider groups negotiate with payers in creating and maintaining provider networks. Where providers in a network do not share financial risk through capitation or substantial withholds or if the network does not demonstrate substantial clinical integration, the network may be considered an alliance of competitors and members may not share pricing information. Complex methods of communicating with payers have evolved to avert violations, but the guidelines must be strictly followed to avoid legal exposure.

Complaints about anti-competitive behavior can be brought by private parties or by the government. Violations of anti-trust laws can result in both civil and criminal penalties. Civil penalties include monetary damages, which may include treble damages equal to three times the actual amount of the injury. Civil actions may also result in the award of injunctions where the court orders the defendant to cease the offending behavior and payment of litigation costs. Violation of antitrust laws constitute a criminal felony, punishable by fines and/or imprisonment and loss of license. Investigations of health maintenance organizations and employer coalitions engaged in such behavior in the 1990s has encouraged the government to engage in an aggressive campaign to control fraud and abuse as well.

Health Care Fraud and Abuse

A significant percentage of the national health care costs is attributable to fraud and abuse, by some estimates as much as 10% (Roeder & Sledge, 1996). Fraud is defined under the Medicare regulations as "an intentional deception or misrepresentation made by a person with the knowledge that the deception could result in some unauthorized benefit to himself or some other person" (Code of Federal Regulations, 1995). Abuse occurs when a party delivers a service, but claims reimbursement for a more extensive service than that actually delivered or makes separate claims for component parts of the service delivered (unbundling) when the service should have been billed as one comprehensive service (Davies & Jost, 1998). Fraud and abusive practices are prohibited by countless federal and state laws with penalties ranging from civil damages to fines and imprisonment. Prosecuting health care fraud and abuse has become a top priority for federal, state, and local regulators. Since 1992, there has been a 200% increase in the number of criminal health care cases filed, and every U. S. Attorney's office now has a health care fraud coordinator (Curran & Wallance, 1997). Ferreting out health care fraud and abuse (now the number two priority of some governmental agencies, second only to violent crime) was significantly strengthened by the passage of Title II of the Health Insurance Portability and Accountability Act (HIPPA). The enforcement provisions of this act created a new criminal statutory scheme with more severe penalties, including a forfeiture provision that authorizes the court to impose forfeiture of property derived directly or indirectly from the commission of an offense.

These provisions, added to the arsenal of other laws and penalties, are designed to crack down on health care criminals. But while some providers do knowingly abuse the system, many unwitting physicians stumble into problems without realizing they are doing anything wrong. These providers simply do not understand the ever-changing landscape of the medical reimbursement system. As new laws are passed and enforcement efforts increase, the net to snare violators is cast more and more broadly. Unlike most criminal sanctions which require willfulness or intent, many health care providers find themselves ensnared by provisions that impose a less onerous standard of "know' or "should have known." For instance, Title II of HIPPA mandates that any individuals or entities who have been convicted of a felony relating to health care fraud in connection with Medicare or Medicaid be excluded from Medicare and Medicaid for at least five years. Title II also authorizes discretionary authority to exclude an individual with a "direct or indirect ownership or control interest in a sanctioned entity" if the individual "knew or should have known" of the wrongdoing without regard to his or her actual involvement (United States Code, Section 42). With this expansive language, arguably a passive investor or outside director of a health care provider group could be effectively barred from the health care industry for failure to take steps to detect or deter a company's health care fraud (Curran & Wallance, 1997). Although certainly not an exhaustive list of fraud and abuse violations, false claims, anti-kickback statutes, and self-referrals are among the areas of greatest risk for most health care providers.

In health care, the term false claims incorporates several types of wrongdoing including bills for services not performed, improperly coded, not provided by the person claiming to have provided them, or provided unnecessarily (Jost, 1994). The False Claims Act of 1863 (FCA), while certainly not confined to health care, prohibits false claims against federal programs, which of course includes Medicare. Claims may be brought by the government or by private individuals on behalf of the government. The right of a private person to prosecute a false claim against the government is granted by a provision known as qui tam. In other words, a qui tam lawsuit is brought to action by a private individual and the state prosecutes it with the likelyhood that the individual gets a percentage of the award. This provision allows the individual, called a relator, to recover a portion of the proceeds of the action or settlement. A typical award would be 15% of the proceeds. Large recoveries have proven to be very enticing to disgruntled employees and competitors, who are the source of a large number of qui tam suits. Whether driven by revenge, greed, or a good faith interest in righting a wrong, relators in qui tam suits are very threatening to providers because they have knowledge of the business and access to records and information of the defendant.

Criminal liability under the FCA requires proof that a defendant knowingly presented a false or fraudulent claim for payment to the government. The term "knowing" includes actual knowledge of the falsity or reckless disregard for the truth. Violations of the FCA may subject a provider to criminal penalties including large fines and imprisonment. Civil penalties can also be assessed under a less onerous standard of proof of "know, or should have known," and under agency principles, physician providers are also liable for acts of their employees. Therefore, if a physician's office submits false claims, even without the direct knowledge of the physician, the physician will typically be liable for civil damages. Civil penalties can amount to $2,000 per item or service plus assessments for two times the amount claimed. Civil penalties also include exclusion from Medicare and Medicaid programs. Because Medicare and Medicaid comprise such a significant portion of reimbursement for most medical practices, exclusion from those programs may very well be a career ending event for many providers or plans.

Exclusion from Medicare and Medicaid programs and criminal penalties may also be imposed for violation of the anti-kickback laws. The federal anti-kickback law prohibits the knowing or willful payment, offering, solicitation, or receipt of remuneration in return for referrals in connection with any service that may be paid for by Medicare or Medicaid (Anti-kickback Law, 1988). For example, under traditional fee-for-service, physicians might receive kickbacks for referring patients to certain specialists, while under managed care plans specialists paid on a capitated basis might pay kick-backs to gatekeepers for withholding referrals. While these are straight-forward examples, in the managed care environment other violations can be unintended and unclear. Because there was so much uncertainty as to what actions might violate the broad prohibitions of the anti-kickback statutes, the Office of the Inspector General has issued its final rules revising safe harbors for managed care plans under the anti-kickback law. One of these safe harbors protects certain enrollee incentives offered by health plans to encourage use of in-network providers; a second applies to price reductions offered to health plans by contract health care providers. Even though the revised safe harbors have clarified some ambiguity, there is still ample uncertainty about how to structure many managed care arrangements without violating the anti-kickback prohibitions.

Self-referrals can also be a potential stumbling block for providers. Prohibitions to self-referrals are found in laws commonly referred to as the Stark laws—Stark I and Stark II. Stark I prohibits physicians from referring Medicare patients for clinical laboratory services to entities with which they or an immediate family member have ownership or an investment interest. This prohibition does not apply to in-office laboratory services or services provided under the personal supervision and billed by the referring physician or another physician in the same practice. Competing physicians who practice separately may not, however, share in the overhead of the operation of a laboratory, even when the physicians practice in the same building.

Stark II, which took affect January 1, 1995, expanded the Stark I prohibitions to include a number of "designated health services" and Medicaid services. Some of the services included under Stark II are radiology, physical and occupational therapy, prescription drugs and home health, and hospital services. Final regulations on Stark II are still pending, and they will undoubtedly affect referral and utilization activities of many physicians. Under the proposed regulations, a claim that violates the Stark requirements also violates the FCA and other fraud and abuse statutes thus subjecting the providers to another layer of civil and criminal penalties (Caeser, 1997).

As discussed earlier in this chapter, enforcement of health care fraud and abuse was strengthened with the passage of HIPPA, which became effective June 1, 1997. One goal of HIPPA was to target health care fraud and abuse, armed with greater focus, better funding, and harsher penalties. The Act created new programs to oversee Medicare, encourage the reporting of violations, give guidance to providers, and enhance penalties for violations. But one of the most significant provisions in HIPPA is found in the criminal law provision defining "health care fraud" as the knowing and willful attempt or execution to defraud "any health care benefit program." This language indicates that abuses are no longer confined to Medicare and Medicaid, but now apply to all benefit plans. This makes the reach of the fraud and abuse laws more broad than ever and with the addition of stronger penalties greatly increases the legal exposure for providers. The single provision that is likely to have the greatest impact on fraud and abuse enforcement efforts, however, provides for increased funding for health care enforcement by creating a trust fund maintained by proceeds from asset forfeitures.

These developments underscore the need for providers to take great care in submitting claims and contracting with other providers and managed care networks. The importance of developing comprehensive internal compliance programs cannot be overstated. The benefits of these programs are twofold. First, they provide a defined internal mechanism to ensure compliance with the complicated laws and regulations. Second, they offer some measure of protection if violations do occur because federal regulators have stated that when sanctions are imposed, consideration will be given to the fact the provider did have a compliance program indicating an intention to comply with the law and effort to use proper billing practices.

In addition to compliance programs, another way of proactively avoiding legal issues is to create an environment that has a strong ethical culture.

ETHICAL STANDARDS FOR THE BUSINESS OF HEALTH CARE

Physician leaders are uniquely positioned to influence ethical awareness in the workplace. Understanding the basic underpinnings of ethical theory and empirical research in ethics will give physician leaders a grounding in the ethical implications of their decisions.

Westgaard (1988, p. 17) explains the need for caveats that allow us to expand our ethical awareness:

> "The basic value which identifies true professionals is their drive to give full measure and do their best. To do less, to settle for a half-measure, is disrespectful of oneself, others, and the profession. Failure to establish ethical controls results in unfair competition, misunderstandings with clients and risks of scandals to the profession. Any professional must seek to lessen the possibility of unfair competition practices by establishing and adhering to ethical guidelines."

Ethical Standards Help Us Create an Ethical Climate

There is an another equally compelling reason for physician leaders to expand their ethical understanding. Only by being aware of ethical considerations oneself can a professional help the practice of medicine. Physician leaders ought to be able to help health care organizations recognize that the ethical climate in an organization is one of the environmental factors that impact performance and productivity. For instance, the motivation of health care employees can be negatively influenced by:

- inconsistent application of policies
- lack of concern for the rights or safety of the individual
- failure of the organization to comply with the law
- misrepresentation to suppliers or clients.

Likewise, withholding information or establishing unrealistic expectations in an attempt to gain control or power are unethical acts that damage performance output (Dean, 1993). This can have a major impact on the results of the process. Operating from the premise that creating and maintaining an ethical environment ought to be within the mission of an effective organization, as well as being a good business practice, physician leaders have a context for addressing ethical problems in a straightforward manner. They can suggest the need to examine the ethical congruence of the different functions, policies, and levels of the organization to assure an environment that encourages exemplary performance. Another important expectation is to help the organization recognize how a solution implemented at one level will impact the organization as a whole. This is one of our ethical responsibilities.

Ethics Officers

A new trend in business and industry worth noting here is that of a new function known as ethicist or ethical officer (EO). Chief Executive Officers and other corporate executives are now expected to use ethicists who provide ethical advice. This is similar to a Medical Ethical Committee who would be consulted on a point of ethics regarding the practice of medicine. Here, an EO would be consulted on an issue of business practice. According to Hoffman (personal correspondence with Kamm, 1991), "our best estimate is that between fifteen and twenty-five percent of the Fortune 500 have someone to oversee corporate ethics . . . because the position of ethics office is so new, there is no book on the shelf to tell them what to do." The percentage has surely increased with the advent of required ethics courses in MBA and EMBA curriculums.

What is required of an ethicist or ethical officer? Gustafson (1991), as found in Dean (1993), indicates the following standards:

- Ethicists must understand the ethical/moral concepts of:
    —utilitarian ways to evaluate benefits and harms of a decision
    —rights, rules, responsibilities from the formalistic tradition
    —social justice and social contract literature
    —the criteria for sound moral arguments
    —the historical ethical traditions stemming from philosophy and religion
    —the subject matter at issue, e.g., taxation policies, selection procedures, etc.
- Ethicists should point out the strengths and weaknesses of these ethical underpinnings with regard to practical choice.

A corporate ethicist should be concerned with any situation in which there is an actual or potential harm to an individual or group at any and all levels of the organization. The harm may be physical, mental, or economic. It is also a concern when the rights of one individual compete with the rights of another or when rights of different levels of the organization compete with each other. Cooke (1992), as found in Dean (1993), focuses on these situations by raising several questions:

- Is the behavior or anticipated behavior arbitrary or capricious? Does it unfairly single out any individual or group?
- Does the behavior or anticipated behavior violate moral and legal rights of any individual or group?

- Does the behavior or anticipated behavior conform to accepted ethical/moral standards?
- Are there alternative courses of action that are less likely to cause harm?

An ethicist believes that such questions must be raised whenever there is actual or potential harm.

Maclagan (1983) indicates that all professionals should be aware of key ethical issues. Those issues are:

- confidentially
- inappropriate requests
- intellectual property
- truth in claims
- organizational versus individual needs
- customer and user participation
- conflicts of interest
- personal biases
- individual and population differences
- appropriate interventions
- intervention consequences
- pricing fairly
- using power.

Administrators typically look at the financial data collected, transform it into information to be used in decision-making, and judge the consequences of using that information. This approach often leads to an ends-justifies-the-means logic that may fail to provide an ethical climate. This logic is called consequential, utilitarian, or goal-oriented management (Keeley, 1979; Krupp, 1961; Pfeffer, 1978). But there are two sides to the story (Dean, 1993).

Knowledge of the two sides of ethics will heighten our ethical awareness and decision making capability. This in turn will provide an additional way to help our client organizations. The following provides a review of the key ethical theories so we can increase our ethical awareness and knowledge.

Two Traditional Sides of Business Ethics

Normative ethical theories that there are various ways to classify decisions have been suggested for centuries, beginning with the pre-Socratics in the sixth century BC. There are two basic categories: consequentialism (results) and intentionality (rules). Each of these categories represents a vantage point regarding the purposes and processes of ethical decision making (Dean, 1993).

Results (Consequentialism or Utilitarianism)

Consequentialism examines the net benefit produced for all stakeholders, primarily the stakeholders who hold stock in a company. It evaluates an action in terms of the efficiency and effectiveness of its consequence (Arthur Andersen & Co, 1992). Thus, the rightness or wrongness of an action is determined by its consequences. People's rights, duty, their sense of justice, and their values are not of primary consideration, just the consequences (Bentham, 1979; Mill, 1863/1957; Sidgwick, 1874/1966). "The end justifies the means" is one of the expressions used to describe consequentialism (Dean, 1993).

Consequentialism suggests planning, calculating, decision making, and evaluation can encourage creativity, innovation, productivity, and entrepreneurship. It should result in the best possible consequences for the organization's goals. These consequences maximize the satisfaction of the organization's constituencies, usually the owners. One question that a consequentialist asks is, "Which action will produce the greatest good?" To answer this question, he or she must also ask which action produces the greatest good for whom. In answering the latter half of this question, the field of consequentialism can be divided into two areas: utilitarianism and egoism (Dean, 1993).

As Dean (1993) and Ferrell & Fraedrich (1991) suggest, utilitarianism examines consequences to others. Business is most comfortable with utilitarian theory because it traces its roots to Adam Smith (1776), the father of modern economics. Yet, Adam Smith wrote about utilitarianism and, though most business people do not realize it, he wrote persuasively about duty and justice in *The Theory of Moral Sentiment* in 1759, seventeen years before *Wealth of Nations* was published. Utilitarian theory was further defined by the research of Jeremy Bentham (1748-1832) and John Stuart Mill (1806-1873). These two men used utilitarian standards to evaluate and criticize the social and political systems of their time period. As a result, utilitarianism is commonly associated with social improvement (Shaw & Barry, 1989).

There are a variety of factors, in addition to social improvement and avoiding harm, that make utilitarianism attractive to business and industry today. Some factors are that it:

- provides a basis for formulating and testing policies
- provides an objective way of resolving conflicts of self-interest
- recognizes the four primary stakeholders: owners, employees, customers, and society
- provides the latitude in moral decision making that organizations seem to need (Dean, 1993; Shaw & Barry, 1989).

Bentham is well known for his "greatest happiness" principle. His concept of the greatest good for the greatest number of people is based on the outcome that produces the most happiness for all persons (Dean, 1993).

"The reason Bentham was so interested in this principle is that it provided the rationale for advocating reform of laws and institutions that protected only the traditionally preferred classes of citizens, while dealing harshly with others. Tradition, he felt, often discriminated, but the greatest happiness principle did not; it gave equal weight to every individual" (Brady, 1990, p. 39).

An additional appeal of utilitarianism is its emphasis on efficiency. "Efficiency is a means to higher profits and to lower prices, and the struggle to be maximally profitable seeks to obtain maximum production from limited economic resources" (Beauchamp & Bowie, 1988, p. 26).

Examples of utilitarianism in today's business and industry are:

- cost benefit analysis
- environmental impact studies
- the majority vote
- product comparisons for consumer information
- tax laws
- consumer behavior in the free market (Brady, 1990).

Each of these activities determines the worth of a situation by evaluating the consequences for all persons affected by the action.

From the overall vantage point of consequentialism, it becomes easy to overlook the ethics of the means (the behavior) that are used to achieve the actual ends (the accomplishment). In addition, the long-term consequences are often not taken into account. Bok (1980) suggests that decision makers should periodically assess managerial strategies to be sure that all of the organization's constituencies are being considered, not just the owners (Dean, 1993).

Rules (Intentionality or Deontology)

Intentionality is referred to as deontology by ethicists. It is defined as a moral philosophy that "focuses on the rights of individuals and on the intentions associated with a particular behavior" (Ferrell & Fraedrich, 1991, p.45). A deontologist believes that the moral rightness or wrongness of an action takes precedence over and, for the most part, can be judged independently of the consequences (Wagner, 1991). Whereas the consequentialist conducts an ends analysis in determining ethical alternatives, the deontologist is more concerned with a means evaluation (Dean, 1993). In deontology, what matters is the nature of the act in question, not just its results (Shaw & Barry, 1989). Such actions as keeping a personal promise, abiding by the terms of a contract, repaying a debt, and ensuring fairness of distribution are considered "right" regardless of the consequences that follow (Beauchamp & Bowie, 1988).

Deontology emphasizes the importance of duty and motives in making and acting upon ethical decisions (Beauchamp & Bowie, 1988). A person's behavior is important as it binds us to (or prohibits us from) the action (Wagner, 1991). It provides a standard of behavior through rules. Common deontological practices in business and industry include:

- distributing benefits and profit equitably
- upholding constitutional rights
- making decisions based on doctrines or codes
- specifying hours of operation
- wearing uniforms (Brady, 1990).

Deontological practices and standards "attempt to generate a total set of expectations that seem to preserve important relations and values" (Brady, 1990, p. 22). Establishing standards of intentionality, however, does not guarantee ethical outcomes. What it does do is provide the individual with a set of guidelines to follow in ethical decision making (Dean, 1993). Many ethical theories have been developed from the vantage point of deontology. As cited in Dean (1993), the most prominent is reason-based ethics as explained by Kant.

Immanuel Kant (1965) pursued moral principles that do not rest on consequences and that define actions as inherently right or wrong, apart from circumstantial factors. In accordance with deontological theory, Kant believed that moral rules were a result of reason alone and that reason guided our moral beliefs (Shaw & Barry, 1989). His idea of pure reason recognized the "possibility of discovering and knowing moral laws or principles without necessarily liking them or experiencing them, but just by recognizing their authenticity" (Brady, 1990, p. 49). For example, a statement such as "Lying is wrong" may be morally right whether a person likes it or not. In other words, it is unconditionally necessary to tell the truth regardless of the consequences. Telling the truth inherently possesses ethical worth.

Kant's theory, called the categorical imperative, is composed of three basic principles.

1. *The Principle of Universality.* An action is morally right for a person in a certain situation if and only if the person's reason for carrying out the action is a reason that he or she would be willing to have every person act on, in any similar situation. (Velasquez, 1992) In other words, if one is applying the principle of universibility, one must be willing to have his or her action become a universal law for others to follow in similar situations. One rule of thumb that is commonly associated with this principle is to ask yourself: "Would I feel comfortable discussing this action on *60 Minutes* or in front of my grandmother?".

2. *The Principle of Reversibility.* The person's reasons for acting must be reasons that he or she would be willing to have all others use, even as a basis of how he or she is treated by others. (Velasquez, 1992) This golden rule of ethics requires that, in assessing an action, a person ask, "How would I like it if I were treated this way?". If a person would wish the same action on him or herself, then it meets the requirements of the reversibility principle.

3. *The Principle of Respect for Persons.* "Rational creatures should always treat other rational creatures as ends in themselves and never as only a means to an end" (Shaw & Barry, 1989, p. 64). In attempting to meet this requirement, a person must do two things, respect the freedom of others by treating them only as they have consented to be treated and develop each person's capacity to choose freely among alternatives (Velasquez, 1992).

It was Kant's contention that all human beings possess inherent worth and should be treated with the moral dignity to which they are entitled

(Shaw & Barry, 1989). From the perspective of deontology, people act according to such moral duties and rights of the individual. This principle of respect for a person's rights has become a theory in its own standing (Dean, 1993).

When consistency is lacking as rules are applied, an unfair playing ground is created. This can represent a lack of balance between morals and practice. As a result, individuals are disinclined to perform by the rules. They may be less productive, and unethical behavior may become easier to justify. Also, an overemphasis on justice can reduce entrepreneurship, innovation, and productivity.

These two normative vantage points (consequentialism and intentionality) involve us in continuously examining our own sense of right and wrong and revising it as appropriate. With just a basic understanding of each normative vantage point, physician leaders can help their employees view their problems with a wider-angle lens. Social contract theory provides a contextual basis for using these two normative vantage points with an emphasis on the uncoerced, informed consent of those who will be bound by cultural norms and the two vantage points (Donaldson & Dunfee, 1994)

Traditionally, organizations establish corporate credos, ethical codes, and ethical programs (Murphy, 1989). A credo is a statement that declares the organization's values by providing a general set of beliefs and principles. "Most managers report today that the credo has a powerful influence on their decision making. It stands for day to day values" (Sturdivant & Wortzel, 1990, p. 128).

Ethical codes are behavioral guidelines. They reflect and support the ethical values of the organization, clarify expectations, and recognize specific ethical issues. "Ninety percent of Fortune 500 firms and nearly half of smaller firms have ethical codes or codes of conduct that provide specific guidance to employees in functional business areas" (Sturdivant & Wortzel, 1990, p.129).

Codes of ethics are developed for a variety of reasons: to demonstrate commitment of the CEO; maintain public trust and credibility; encourage managerial professionalism; protect against improper employee conduct; define ethical conduct in light of new laws or social standards; or reflect changing corporate structure and culture (Berenbeim, 1987).

Most codes of ethics address three issues:

1. Being a good employee of the organization.

2. Doing nothing unlawful or improper that might harm the organization.
3. Being good to the customer.

Additionally, codes address other issues depending on the needs of the organization:

- Exhibiting standards of personal integrity and professional conduct.
- Prohibiting racial, ethnic, religious, or sexual harassment.
- Reporting questionable, unethical, or illegal activities to the manager.
- Seeking opportunities to participate in community services and political activities.
- Conserving resources and protecting the quality of the environment in areas where the company operates. (Robin, Giallourakis, David, & Moritz, 1989).

Although codes do establish expectations, researchers agree that used in isolation, they have limited effect in promoting an ethical environment (Berenbeim, 1987; Dean, 1992; Dean, 1994; Dean, 1997; Robin et al., 1989). An ethics program needs to be used in conjunction with a corporate credo and ethical code.

Ethics programs most often consist of training events and communications. Some organizations use training to explain the meaning of their credo and ethical guidelines and to discuss the problems of applying those standards (Andrews, 1989). Ethics programs sensitize employees to ethical issues, broaden awareness of code directives, and emphasize the organization's commitment to its ethical principles (Berenbeim, 1987). In fact, training should not be discounted, as it may be a key to establishing consistent business ethics. Training "makes ethical analysis an integral part of the company's decision making process" (Dean, 1992, p. 288).

Health Care Organizational Issues

Obvious organizational issues that present opportunities for physician leaders to lead with ethics include (Cavanagh, Moberg, & Valasquez, 1981):

- employee rights versus due process, privacy
- sexual harassment
- whistle blowing

- misuse of power
- discouraging intrinsic motivation
- selection and placement
- corporate culture
- corporate social responsibility
- agreed upon incentive system versus actual system
- terminations
- organizational structure, design, and politics
- performance appraisals
- drug testing, physical exams
- diversity/discrimination
- planning, policy, control
- government relations
- safety and health issues
- technical development
- foreign payments
- environmental protection
- product safety, reliability
- quality management
- purchasing (gifts, bribes)
- automation, robotics.

A survey of organizations (Perry, Bennet, & Edwards, 1990) indicated the materials and formats most commonly used in ethics training are:

- codes of ethics (79%)
- lectures (63%)
- workshops and seminars (53%)
- case studies (46%)
- films and discussion (41%).

Case studies and discussions have been found most effective. "They give participants a sense of how to analyze and resolve ethical problems in a way that is consistent with the company's code or standards of corporate conduct" (Berenbeim, 1987, p. 18). Moreover, by combining the case study format with the Critical Incident Technique, participants in ethics training actually generate information related to their organization that they can draw on later as they make decisions (Dean, 1992).

CONCLUSION

Physician leaders are uniquely positioned in their health care systems to facilitate the awareness of business law and the value of business ethical standards. Regarding the actual process of making ethical decisions, it is seldom as easy as simply selecting the correct alternative. Although physician leaders will sometimes face choices between obvious right and wrong, extenuating circumstances will usually exist and they'll face choices between one right and another right. Those are the tough choices. With such choices, it is helpful to apply a step-by-step decision–making process. When confronted with choosing between two right alternatives, ethical decisions depend on the decision-making process; the experience, intelligence, and integrity of the decision maker; and balancing the ethical tensions in a moral free space (T. Donaldson and T.W. Dunfee, personal communication, Wharton Ethics Program, 1998). Sometimes training and coaching can both enhance the decision-making process and enrich the experience of the decision maker (Dean, 1993). Most, however, contain the same basic processes represented in Werhane's (1992) seven-step process for ethical decision making.

Werhane's model has seven steps in the process (Dean, 1993):

1. *Identify the relevant facts*
   Key factors that shape the situation and influence ethical issues must be identified.

2. *Define the ethical issues*
   All issues related to the situation must be identified and the ethical issues separated from the non-ethical issues. Issues may be identified at all levels of the organization.

3. *Identify the primary stakeholders*
   Those individuals and groups involved in the situation that will be affected by a decision are the primary stakeholders. The impact of a decision on them must be considered.

4. *Determine the possible alternatives*
   All alternative interventions need to be identified.

5. *List the ethical implications of each of the alternatives*
   Each alternative needs to be evaluated according to ethical theories (Utilitarianism, Deontology) and the impact on the stakeholders.

6. *List the practical constraints*
Any factors that might limit the implementation of alternatives or render it too difficult or risky must be identified.

7. *Determine which actions should be taken*
After weighing the information provided in steps one through six, an alternative needs to be selected and an implementation strategy identified.

GLOSSARY

antitrust laws. a series of laws passed to limit anticompetitive behavior in almost all businesses, industries, and professions in the United States.

market share. a firm or group's fractional share of the total market. Market may consist of product or service market and geographic market.

messenger model. a messenger is used to ferry information back and forth between the payer and each network participant in order to avoid the sharing of price information directly among competing providers. New guidelines have expanded the role of the messenger.

per se violation. a restraint of trade considered inherently anti-competitive and deemed illegal without further inquiry.

price fixing. any agreement with the purpose of effect of raising, depressing, fixing, or stabilizing prices.

relevant market. There are two kinds of relative markets. 1. Product or service market includes substitute products or services that are interchangeable with the products or services in question. 2. Geographic market includes the territory in which the group sells its product or service.

restraint of trade. when two or more competitors enter into a contract, combination, or conspiracy to unreasonably interfere with competition.

treble damages. damages equal to three times the actual amount of the injury.

SELECTED READINGS FOR HEALTH CARE LAW

Annals of Health Law, The False Claims Act: An Old Weapon with New Firepower Is Aimed at Health Care Fraud, Ryan, D., Vol. 4, 1995.

The Antitrust Health Care Handbook, Antitrust Issues Facing Health Care Providers, Section of Antitrust Law, American Bar Association, 1993.

Fundamentals of Health Law, Hastings, D., Luce, G., and Wynstra, N., National Health Lawyers Association.

Health Law Handbook, Gosfield, A., West Group, 1997 & 1998.

Managed Care Contracting, Concepts and Applications for the Health Care Executive, Conrad, D., Bonney, R., Sachs, M., and Smith, R., Health Administration Press, Chicago, IL 1996.

Managed Care: Placebo or Wonder Drug for Health Care Fraud and Abuse?, Davies, S. and Jost, T., Available: http://www.lawsch.uga.edu/-galawrev/vol31/davies.html

Medicare Medicaid Safe Harbors Handbook, Do's and Don'ts For Joint Ventures and Other Healthcare Business Arrangements, Cacioppo, P., 1993.

Physician's Survival Guide: Legal Pitfalls and Solutions, The National Health Lawyers Association and The American Medical Association, 1991.

SELECTED JOURNALS IN BUSINESS ETHICS

Some organizations and societies in business ethics are included so that ethical officers in health care organizations dealing with ethical issues are aware of some of the resources available to them.

Business Ethics Magazine
Business Ethics
1107 Hazeltine Boulevard, Suite 530
Chaska, MN 55318
612-448-8864

Business Ethics Quarterly
Patricia H. Werhane, Editor-in-Chief
Ronald Duska, Executive Director
Darden Graduate School of Business Administration
University of Virginia
Charlottesville, VA 22906
804-924-4840
610-526-1387

Business and Professional Ethics Journal
Center for Applied Psychology
240 "A" Arts and Science Building
University of Florida
Gainesville, FL 32611
904-392-2084

Business and Society Review
Management Reports, Inc.
25-13 Old Kings Highway, Suite 107
Darien, CT 06820

Ethics: Easier Said than Done
Josephson Institute
310 Washington Boulevard, Suite 104
Marina Del Ray, CA 90292
213-306-1868

Ethikos
Ethikos, Inc.
799 Broadway, Suite 541
New York, NY 10003
212-228-7537

Journal of Business Ethics
Kluwer Academic Publishers Group
P.O. Box 358
Accord Station
Hingham, MA 02018-0358
617-871-6600

The International Journal of Applied Philosophy
Philosophy Documentation Center
Bowling Green University
Bowling Green, OH 43403-0189
1-800-444-2419

The International Journal of Value-based Management
Institute for Business and Management Ethics
Hagan School of Business
Iona College
New Rochelle, NY 10901
914-633-2256

Business Ethics: A European Review
Business Ethics Centre
King's College
Strand
London, WC2R 2LS
071-873-2587

REFERENCES

Andrews, K.B. (1989). Ethics in practice. *Harvard Business Review, 67*, 99–104.

Anti-kickback Law. (1988). 42 U.S.C., Section 1320a-7b(b).

Arthur Andersen & Co. (1992). *Ethics for managers: Instructors guide.* St. Charles, IL: Author.

Baron, D. (1991). *Business and its environment.* Englewood Cliffs, NJ: Prentice Hall.

Beauchamp, T.L., & Bowie, N.E. (1988). *Ethical theory and business* (3rd ed.). Englewood Cliffs, NJ: Prentice Hall.

Bentham, J. (1979). *An introduction to the principle of morals and legislation.* London: Athlone Press. (Originally published in 1789)

Berenbeim, R.E. (1987). *Corporate ethics* (Research Report #900). New York: The Conference Board.

Brady, F.N. (1990). *Ethical managing: Rules and results.* New York: Macmillan Publishing USA.

Caesar, N. (1997, May). New Stark II rules on referrals will further restrict medical practices. *Managed Care Magazine* [online]. Available: http://www.managedcaremag.com/archiveMC/9705/9705.legal.shtml

Cavanagh, G.F., Moberg, D.J., & Velasquez, M. (1981). The ethics of organizational politics. *Academy of Management Review, 66*, 363–374.

Chicago Board of Trade v. United States, 246 U.S. 231 (1918).

Code of Federal Regulations, 42 C.F.R., Section 455.2 (1995).

Cohen, J. (1997, May 12). Changes in antitrust guidelines affect physician networks and IPAs, *South Florida Business Journal* [online]. Available: http://cgi.amcity.com/southflorida/stories/051297/focus2.html

Cooke, R.A. (1992). *Ethics in business: A perspective.* St. Charles, IL: *Business Ethics Program,* Arthur Andersen & Co.

Curran, P., & Wallance, G. (1997, January 20). Title II of the Health Insurance Portability and Accountability Act makes civil and administrative sanctions for fraud harsher. *The National Law Journal,* B5.

Davies, S., & Jost, T. (1998). Managed care: Placebo or wonder drug for health care fraud and abuse? [online]. Available: http://www.lawsch.uga.edu/-galawrev/vol31/davies.html.

Dean, P.J. (1992). Making codes of ethics 'real.' *Journal of Business Ethics, 11,* 285–291.

Dean, P.J. (1993). A selected review of the underpinnings of ethics for human performance technology professionals part 1 and 2. *Performance Improvement Quarterly, 6,* 3–49.

Dean, P.J. (1994, February). Some basics about ethics. *Performance and Instruction,* 36–45, 49.

Dean, P.J. (1997). Examining the profession and the practice of business ethics. *Journal of Business Ethics, 16,* 1637–1649.

Donaldson, T., & Dunfee, T.W. (1994). Toward a unified conception of business ethics: integrative social contracts theory. *Academy of Management Review, 19*(2), 252–284.

False Claims Act. (1863). 31 U.S.C., Sections 3729–3732 (1988 & Supplement 1993).

Ferrell, O.C., & Fraedrich, J. (1991). *Business ethics: ethical decision making and cases.* Boston, MA: Houghton Mifflin.

Gustafson, J.M. (1991). Ethics: An American growth industry. *The Key Reporter, 56,* 6–11.

Jost, T. (1994). Medicare and medicaid false claims: Prohibitions and sanctions. *Annals of Health Law, 3,* 41.

Kant, I. (1965). *The metaphysical elements of justice* (J. Ladd, trans). New York: Library of Liberal Arts. (Original published in 1785)

Keeley, M. (1979). *Justice versus effectiveness in organizational evaluation.* Paper presented at the annual meeting of the Academy of Management, Atlanta, Georgia.

Klein, S.A. (1998). Group mergers face FTC scrutiny. *American Medical News, 41,* 1.

Krupp, S. (1961). *Patterns of organizational analysis.* New York: Holt, Rinehart & Winston.

Maclagan, P.W. (1983). The concept of responsibility: Some implications for organizational behavior and development. *Journal of Management Studies, 20,* 411–423.

Mann, A., & Roberts, B. (1997). *Smith and Roberson's business law* (10th ed.). St. Paul, MN: West Publishing Co.

Mill, J.S. (1957). *Utilitarianism.* Indianapolis, IN: Bobbs-Merrill. (Original published in 1863)

Murphy, P.E. (1989, Winter). Creating ethical corporate structures. *Sloan Management Review,* 81–87.

Perry, D., Bennet, K., & Edwards, G. (1990). *Ethics policies and programs.* Washington, DC: Ethics Resource Center.

Pfeffer, J. (1978). The micropolitics of organizations. In M.W. Meyer et al (Eds.), *Environments and organizations* (pp. 29–50). San Francisco, CA: Jossey-Bass, Publishers.

Robin, D., Giallourakis, M., David, F.R., & Moritz, T.E. (1989). A different look at codes of ethics. *Business Horizons, 32,* 66–73.

Roeder, K.H., & Sledge, S.K. (1996, Oct. 14). Health care law. *National Law Journal,* B5.

Shaw, W., & Barry, V. (1989). *Moral issues in business* (4th ed.). Belmont, CA: Wadsworth.

Sherman Antitrust Act. (1890). 15 U.S.C., Section 2.

Sidgwick, H. (1966). *The methods of ethics.* New York: Dover. (Original published in 1874)

Smith, A. (1759). *Essays philosophical and literary.* London: Ward, Lock, & CO.

Smith, A. (1937). *The wealth of nations.* New York: The Modern Library. (Original published in 1776).

Sturdivant, F.D., & Wortzel, H.V. (1990). *Business and society: A managerial approach* (4th ed.). Boston, MA: Irwin.

United States Code, 42 U.S.C. 1320a-7(b)(15).

Velasquez, M.G. (1992). *Business ethics: Concepts and cases* (3rd ed.). Englewood Cliffs, NJ: Prentice Hall.

Wagner, M.F. (1991). *An historical introduction to moral philosophy.* Englewood Cliffs, NJ: Prentice Hall.

Werhane, P.H. (1992, July). *Corporate moral and social responsibility.* Paper presented at Ethics Practice and Teaching Workshop, Colorado Springs, CO.

Westgaard, O. (1988). *A credo for performance technologists.* Western Springs, IL: International Board of Standards for Training, Performance and Instruction.

PART IV

Turning Data Into Information Using Technology

Learning in a Variable World: Statistics and Decision Making for Physician Leaders

David L. Sylwester

TABLE OF CONTENTS

EXECUTIVE SUMMARY

We are living in what is commonly termed the information age. In our computer oriented society, massive amounts of data are collected and are available to assist in decision making. Indeed, failing to take advantage of data sources puts a manager at a critical disadvantage relative to the competition. Statistics is a collection of concepts and tools that can assist the modern manager in collecting, analyzing, and interpreting data. This includes methods of designing studies to enable issues to be addressed using samples of data, thereby saving time and money. Finally statistics has limitations which management must be aware of lest the manager jump to conclusions not supported by the data. In short, it is essential that an executive MBA program customized for physician leaders include statistics as an integral part of decision making.

INTRODUCTION

Statistics and Medical Practice

Statistics in the broad sense is a body of knowledge comprising concepts and methods for learning from experience. This includes

- methods of designing efficient studies
- guidelines on carrying out studies and collecting data
- techniques for summarizing and analyzing data
- interpreting the analysis results

There are many steps between the formulation of the study question and the final conclusion. The science of statistics touches on most of these steps.

At some point in a physician's career, he or she begins to notice that decisions on patient care are not made with certainty but rather with a hedge based on experience and on reports in the medical literature. "Your symptoms might be due to R, so I think we should order tests X, Y and Z, just to be safe." Or instead it might be "Your symptoms are probably not due to R, so we can avoid for the moment ordering the expensive tests X, Y and Z. Take two aspirin and call me in the morning." The physician has come to realize that variation and uncertainty come with the job, but also that the uncertainty can be reduced through collecting additional information coupled with an understanding of the human body.

Statistics is now an essential part of experimentation in the basic medical sciences, epidemiology, and clinical studies. The use of statistical concepts and methods to design and analyze experiments in the basic medical sciences was an easy sell. Treatment levels could be selected and responses could usually be reliably measured. Such studies were a straightforward application of planned agricultural experiments which had seen great advances through the pioneering work of the British statistician, R. A. Fisher, in the first half of this century.

At the other extreme are epidemiologic studies relying on observational data without randomized assignment of treatments to participants. For example, the National Halothane Study of the 1960s sought to determine if halothane, a very popular anesthetic, carried excess risk of death due to liver damage. Data from 850,000 surgeries with 17,000 deaths were collected and analyzed. It was important to adjust the anesthetic-specific death rates for other variables, such as age, physical status, and type of operation. The conclusion was that halothane did not carry excess mortality risk compared to other anesthetics. This large, expensive, and very important study could not have been accomplished without extensive use of statistical tools for the analysis. An easily readable account of this study is found in Tanur et al (1977) where the National Research Council's full report is referenced.

More recently, the medical community has come to realize the value of statistics in reaching reliable conclusions in clinical studies. Many of these studies seek to minimize (hidden) biases by using randomized double-blind designs. Study sizes may be small (20 patients) or huge. The 1954 field trial of the Salk poliomyelitis vaccine involved over a million young children. It is common (even expected) that journal articles reporting medical studies include a description of statistical methods used, give confidence intervals, and that numerical results are "blessed" with P-values.

The *New England Journal of Medicine* has published many articles on the use of statistics in medicine. These have been conveniently packaged in a book edited by John C. Bailar III and Frederick Mosteller (1992).

Statistics and Management

If one hopes to be successful in "management by the numbers," it is evident that the numbers must be correct and relevant to the issue at hand. Modern managers depend on the data collected by the Census Bureau, the National Bureau of Economic Research, and other agencies to be accurate and timely. Furnished with accurate and relevant data, planners are better able to predict future needs in housing, public facilities, durable goods, and financial markets.

Corporations carry out their own surveys to assess the market potential of new products and possible effects of price changes of existing products. Sample selection methods and tested interview procedures and questionnaires enable reliable information to be obtained with relatively small sample sizes. Indeed, a manager may lose credibility by approving a larger-than-needed survey to decide an issue. (One wonders who was responsible for predicting the success of New Coke.)

Within a company, there are many arenas where statistics is used. Statistical optimization methods are used to aide in decisions on locating plants and warehouses to minimize costs in obtaining materials and in shipping to customers. Modern manufacturing operations use statistics as an essential part of quality management programs. One goal in quality management is to identify sources of variation and then modify procedures to reduce or neutralize the variation. Auditors sometimes use sampling to ascertain correctness of stated inventories. Transportation companies use sampling to ascertain how receipts should be divided among several carriers that jointly transported some cargo or some passengers. In the human resources (HR) department, tests are used to predict a candidate's suitability for a specific job. It is important for the HR director to have an appreciation for the degree of reliability of such selection methods.

In most instances, managers do not collect or analyze the data themselves. But they do make decisions informed by statistical analysis results. To understand and correctly interpret such results, it is critical for managers to have an understanding of basic statistical concepts and tools.

Chapter Outline

The statistics topics covered in this chapter are divided into three broad areas:

1. Collecting data,
2. Summarizing data,
3. Making inferences from data.

Collecting data

Statistics deals with learning about populations from samples. By population we mean the set of items about which we wish to make a statement. The population of interest may already exist, such as the collection of all households in the service area of a hospital. Or the population may be one that is continuously being created, such as the population of individuals who will use a medical center's MRI scanning services in the next five years. In either case, learning about the population requires the selection of a sample that is representative of the population. Statistics includes procedures for identifying populations and selecting samples that will enable the investigator to make inferences about the population. For experiments with several treatment groups and one or more control variables, the design of the study is an extremely important statistical issue.

Summarizing data

Data in raw form is of limited use. But appropriately summarized, it can be very informative, especially for extremely large data sets. Both graphic and numeric summaries are useful. Graphic summaries include histograms showing how the data is distributed and scatterplots showing how several variables are related. Numeric summaries include means, standard deviations, and percentiles. An essential part of summarizing data is detecting errors (from incorrect recording or from errors in data entry) and adjusting for missing values.

Making inferences from data

Using data to reach conclusions about a population requires jumping from the particular (the sample) to the general (the population). Examples are determining drug dosage levels that are both safe and efficacious, estimating the percent of patients covered by medical insurance and creating a severity score to help parents manage their asthmatic child. Statistical inferences invariably include information related to the uncertainty of the estimate. Examples are standard errors of sample means and estimated slopes, confidence intervals for population parameters and probability values for tests of hypothesis.

The inference step is fraught with opportunities for error. Errors can arise from using a sample that is not representative of the population of interest, collecting biased data due to poorly phrased questionnaire items, and ignoring (through ignorance or laziness) assumptions required for the statistical procedures used to be valid. Errors also arise from an incorrect interpretation of the analysis results through inadequate understanding by the manager making the interpretation.

Each of the broad areas of collecting data, summarizing data, and making inferences will be discussed through examples to highlight some of the statistical issues. Although those issues have technical components to be addressed by technical specialists, they also require input from managers and leaders of the organization. Moreover, if study conclusions are not clearly understood by the organization's leaders, the chances of the study recommendations being implemented are greatly reduced.

COLLECTING DATA

Example 1. Assessing Patient Satisfaction Levels

Suppose you are the CEO of a large acute care medical center and the Board of Directors has requested that you determine the satisfaction level of the patients who use the facilities for at least one night. Since the center furnishes many types of services (room, food, drug dispensing, etc.) you decide to use a questionnaire in a survey of patients.

Here are some statistical issues related to planning and executing the survey to assess patient satisfaction levels:

1. What are the pros and cons of surveying a sample of the patients rather than the entire population?
2. If a sample is to be used, how shall it be selected to be representative of the patient population? Should we sample patients while in their room or as they check out of the hospital? What are the relative merits of a simple random sample, a stratified random sample, a cluster sample, and a convenience sample?
3. How shall the questionnaire be administered: by each patient's nurse, by a trained interviewer, or self-administered?
4. Do we need to pretest the questionnaire? If so, how should this be done?

The questions above are only a few of the many issues to be settled before the data collection begins. These questions have to do with study efficiency and cost (1), bias (2), and reliability (3 and 4). While a physician leader may not have specific answers, he or she needs to be able to understand the questions asked and realize the importance of taking the time and effort to carefully address issues such as those above.

Example 2. Comparing Suppliers

A large outpatient clinic seeks to reduce its inventory of office sup-plies by requiring just-in-time delivery. Three suppliers are under con-sideration. The clinic director plans to sign a long-term purchasing agreement with one or more of the suppliers. How shall the purchasing manager decide which supplier and what specifications shall be put into the agreement?

As usual, the purchasing manager is nervous because the director ex-pects the correct answer in a short time period. He or she starts thinking about how to proceed after talking with a number of staff members who have some previous experience with the suppliers. Here are some statisti-cal questions he or she formulates:

Q1. Is a supplier speedy in average delivery time for one type of supply but slow for another type?

Q2. Even if some supplies have an acceptable average delivery time, might the variation in delivery times be unacceptable?

Q3. How large a sample do we need to have sufficiently precise esti-mates of average delivery times?

Q4. How can we determine if current delivery data is a reliable predic-tor of future performance?

The purchasing manager is faced with a complication since there may be an interaction between supplier and type of supply. That is, the average delivery time for a supplier differs from type to type (Q1). While the aver-age delivery time is certainly a key response variable, the variation around the average (Q2) is also important for smooth operation at the clinic. Both the average and the standard deviation will influence specifications set for delivery times.

An informed physician leader recognizes the critical importance of a feasible study design to accomplish the goals of the study. The physician leader recognizes that delivery specifications will need to reflect the inherent variability in the delivery times (Q2 and Q3). He or she must also specify the level of precision required as well as level of confidence (e.g., 95%) desired (Q3). Finally, the important concept of statistical control used in quality management assists the physician leader in as-certaining if current delivery time data is a reliable predictor of future performance (Q4).

Example 3. Sex Discrimination in Salaries

The board of directors of a large medical laboratory has charged the CEO with responding to claims by some of the female laboratory technicians of discrimination against females in salary levels. The CEO has passed the issue on to the HR director. The HR director carries out an initial investigation and confirms that average salaries for female technicians are indeed less than that for males. But the director notices other differences between the two groups: years employed, current academic degree, age when hired, and academic degree when hired. How can all this data be used to address the important issue of discrimination in salary levels? Some specific statistical questions may be addressed:

- How are the variables (sex, year's employed, academic degree, etc.) related to each other and to salary levels?
- Which variables should be used jointly to describe salary levels?
- Since salaries are not set by an exact formula, how can the women sustain a claim of discrimination?
- If there is discrimination, how should we decide on a fair adjustment amount for each female technician?

At first glance, the problem may appear to be very difficult, if not impossible, to analyze and reach conclusions. The data may have high associations among two or more of the explanatory variables (e.g., age and years employed). The male technicians may differ markedly from their female associates in terms of age, academic degree, etc. Multiple regression analysis may shed light on the claim. Ideally, the HR director has previously seen multiple regression applied to other observational studies such as this one and will direct staff persons to carry out the work.

In all three of the examples above, we have attempted to briefly describe a realistic problem where statistical concepts and tools can make a significant contribution to the solution. But to make this happen requires management with sufficient understanding and appreciation of statistics to direct that the necessary statistical work be done. Since decisions will be made based on subsequent statistical analysis, it is useful for management to be involved in formulating and refining questions such as those posed for the examples above. A physician leader will increase his/her value to the organization by having knowledge of basic statistical concepts and tools.

SUMMARIZING DATA

Example 1. Assessing Patient Satisfaction Levels

The most usual summary of statistical data from surveys consist of reporting simple averages and standard deviations of the primary variables. But much more can be done to gain a better understanding of the differences in satisfaction level among various groups of patients. A useful viewpoint for the management to have is that not all of the variation in response is random. Rather, some of that variation is related to patient characteristics such as age, sex, length of stay, etc. For example, quality of food service may be much more important for those with longer lengths of stay. Such knowledge can assist the physician leader in deciding *where* system improvements need to be made.

An important goal of data summarization is to organize the data so that management can identify the primary sources of variation. This is illustrated in the next example.

Example 2. Comparing Suppliers

To identify possible sources of variation we report the average and standard deviation of the delivery time for each supplier for each of several types of supplies. Table 13–1 shows some typical numbers for average delivery times in days.

Table 13–1 includes in the bottom row the average delivery time for each type of supply (averaged across the three suppliers) and in the last column the average delivery time for each supplier (averaged across the types of supplies). Note that the column averages are not of interest to us if we intend to contract with a single supplier. The usefulness of the row averages is questionable due to the pattern seen in Figure 13–1. Figure 13–1 shows that the relative ranking of the three suppliers depends on the type of supply under consideration. For kitchen supplies, B is fastest; for cleaning supplies A is fastest; and for office supplies C is fastest. From a managerial point of view, a single supplier may not be the wisest choice. Figure 13–1 is termed an *interaction plot* for it graphically shows that the average delivery time for each type of supply depends on the particular supplier used. That is, there is an interaction between Supplier and Type of Supply.

Table 13–1 Average delivery times (days) for three suppliers.

Supplier	Type of Supply Kitchen	Cleaning	Office	All
A	1.8	1.2	2.1	1.7
B	1.2	1.9	1.7	1.6
C	2.4	2.1	1.5	2.0
All	1.8	1.7	1.8	1.8

To determine if current delivery time data is a reliable predictor of future performance, we must ascertain if the supplier's delivery process is in statistical control. This will require data over a period of time (including under different weather conditions) so that a *control chart* can be created. For our problem a control chart would simply be a time plot of average delivery times from one supplier. (Because delivery times vary by type of supply, we would create a separate chart for each type.) The plot would also have on it

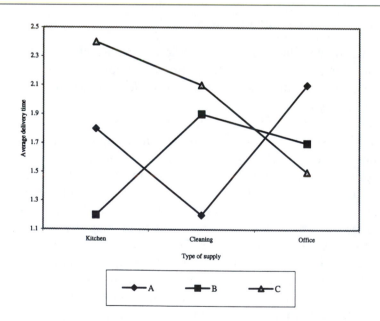

Figure 13–1 Average delivery time (days) for three suppliers (A, B, C) for three types of supplies.

straight lines at the average value and at three standard deviations above and
below the average line. This is illustrated in Figure 14–4.

Example 3. Sex Discrimination in Salaries

This example is perhaps the most complex for it involves six variables
collected on 44 males and 37 females. The scatterplot in Figure 13–2
shows that (no surprise!) salary is closely associated with years employed
for males. Figure 13–3 suggests that salary for males is not closely associated with age when hired. Calculated correlation coefficients are r(salary,
years employed) = 0.77 and r(salary, age when hired) = 0.33.

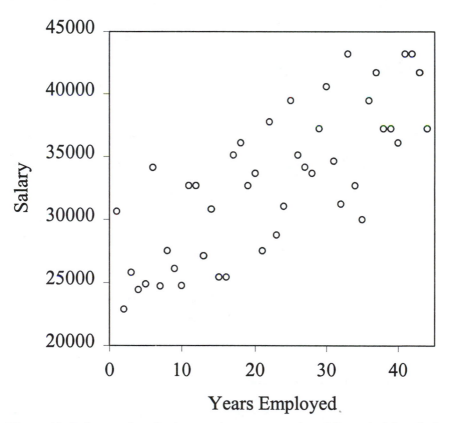

Figure 13–2 Scatterplot of salary against years employed for male lab technicians. *Source:* Data from K.N. Berk and P. Carey, *Data Analysis with Microsoft
Excel,* © 1995, Brooks/Cole Publishing.

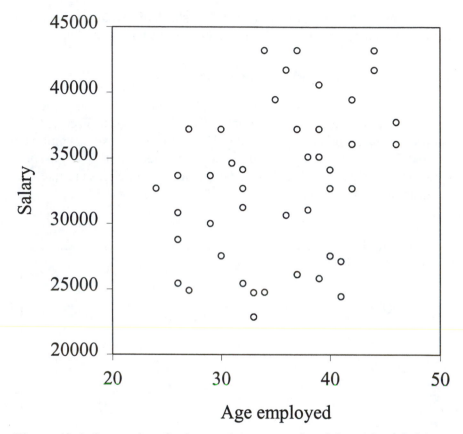

Figure 13–3 Scatterplot of salary against age employed for male technicians. *Source:* Data from K.N. Berk and P. Carey, *Data Analysis with Microsoft Excel,* © 1995, Brooks/Cole Publishing.

Using all the data on males, multiple regression is used to form a prediction equation for male salaries. The equation is

Salary = 12,900 + 744 MS-Hired − 783 Degree + 374 Age-Hired + 606 Years

where MS-Hired = 1 if person had an MS when hired, else MS-Hired = 0; Degree reflects educational level and is coded 1 to 4; and Years is years employed at the lab. Statistical analysis shows that the equation explains about 70% of the variation in male salaries. Plotting the Residuals = (Actual salaries) − (Predicted salaries) for males against Predicted salaries (plot not shown here) shows that about half of the males have salaries above predicted salaries and half have salaries below predicted salaries. In the next section we will use the summary information on males to address the claim of discrimination in salaries for females.

MAKING INFERENCES FROM DATA

Statistical inference consists of making statements about the characteristics of a *population* based on characteristics of a *sample*. These statements are invariably accompanied by an indication of the level of confidence or a probability level. Based on the statements, the physician leader must then decide what action will be taken. (A possible action might be to extend or repeat the study since the essential issues have not been settled with the current data.) We illustrate these ideas using the three examples introduced above.

Example 1. Assessing Patient Satisfaction Levels

Initial analysis may reveal different subgroups of patients with different average levels of satisfaction for particular services. Since the data arise from a sample of patients, it is very useful to know how close the sample average is to the value we would obtain if we had studied the entire hospital patient population (including future patients not yet admitted!). The first step is to determine the standard deviation, which quantifies the variation in the data. The formula for the standard deviation depends on the sampling plan used so it is important that an appropriate sampling plan was used and is known to the analyst. One can then make a confidence interval statement such as "We are 95% confident that between 58% and 76% of our long-stay patients are satisfied with the hospital food". The physician leader may decide that the percent is acceptably high and choose to work on other improvements. Or he or she may decide that the range 76% − 58% = 18% is too large and therefore request more data to be collected to improve the precision of the estimate.

Example 2. Comparing Suppliers

Figure 13–1 suggests that there are differences between suppliers in average delivery times and that the size of the difference may depend on the type of supply. The averages are based on samples of data and thus may not reflect what might be experienced in the long run. Analysis of variance (ANOVA) is a flexible statistical procedure to test whether there are *statistically significant* differences in average delivery time among suppliers, among types of supplies, and whether these two factors interact. The procedure reports a *P-value* which gives the probability of observing results as extreme as that seen in the current data *if in fact the average delivery times are the same for all suppliers, or for all types of supplies*. If the reported probability is small ($P < 0.05$ is frequently taken as small), we say the data are statistically significant (at $P < 0.05$) and reject the original hypothesis of no differences in average delivery times. In that case, confidence intervals are calculated to decide where the actual population differences are.

The analysis above may give us correct results under current delivery conditions but how can we be sure that the present reflects the future? One must look at a control chart, which is a run chart of delivery times over a longer period of time (ideally representing a variety of delivery conditions). If the run chart exhibits "small" variation we conclude that the process is in statistical control and are willing to use present performance to predict future performance. The prediction may tell us that delivery times have too much variation to meet our needs; the supplier will have to reduce that variation. If the run chart exhibits too much variation, then neither the producer nor we can predict future performance with a high degree of reliability. We sign a contract with such a supplier at our peril.

The steps described above are a necessary part of clarifying differences in averages and predictability of future performance. In most cases, actual performance will exhibit variability in outcome. The physician leader must be prepared to consider such variation in specifying performance requirements.

Example 3. Sex Discrimination in Salaries

In the previous section, we presented an equation that described salaries of male technicians using four explanatory variables. The equation is quite useful for it explains about 70% of the variation in male salaries. A careful and thorough statistical analysis would include a search for *outliers*, unusual points that may distort the picture and should be considered for exclusion from the analysis. Not finding any outliers, we can use that equation to assess whether the female lab technicians are paid less than the males after taking into account their individual ages, years employed, and academic degrees. We simply use the equation derived for the males to predict each woman's salary and compare it to her actual salary. Figure 13–4 shows the plot of Residual = (Actual salary) − (Predicted salary) obtained by applying the male equation to the 37 females. These are plotted against the females' predicted salaries. Notice that across all salary levels most of the residuals are negative; the females are generally paid less than males with the same experience profile.

The data support the claim of sexual discrimination in salary levels. The data can also be used to estimate appropriate adjustments for the females. One simply uses the residuals shown in Figure 13–4 since they represent the difference between each female's actual salary and her predicted salary if she were a male with her own experience profile.

The usefulness of the conclusions reached in Example 3 rests on careful planning and execution of data collection, a correct and thorough statistical analysis, and clear communication to management of the implications and limitations of the study. A physician leader will be able to be a more effective leader if he or she understands the basic concepts of statistics and correctly uses data in management activities.

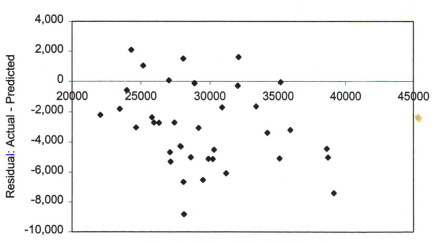

Predicted Salary Using Male Equation

Figure 13–4 Residual plot for female salaries against predicted salaries. Residual = Actual salary − Predicted salary using the male prediction equation. *Source:* Data from K.N. Berk and P. Carey, *Data Analysis with Microsoft Excel,* © 1995, Brooks/Cole Publishing.

CONCLUSION

This chapter has attempted to illustrate through three examples how statistical concepts and tools are used to design efficient studies, collect useful data, analyze data, and interpret the analysis results. In the day-to-day world of decision making the physician leader will find that the careful use of statistics will bring benefits—benefits that will justify the time and cost of careful planning and decision making.

However, political considerations may limit the decision maker's choices. A current example is the ongoing controversy between Congress and the United States Bureau of the Census. The Census Bureau proposes to improve the accuracy of the census count by using statistical sampling as a basis of adjustment of the counts in the 2000 census. While scientifically sound, some congressional persons fear that this could affect apportionment of congressional seats. Currently, it appears that the political concerns of Congress will win the day against the accuracy concerns of the Census Bureau.

A second example is the on-going debate regarding whether women in their 40's should begin to have mammograms as a breast cancer screening device. This has been briefly discussed in Utts (1996). Prior to 1993, both the National Cancer Institute (NCI) and the American Cancer Society (ACS) had recommended that women in their 40's should have mammograms. But in February 1993, the NCI convened an international conference of experts who studied the existing statistical evidence and concluded that there is no reduction in mortality from breast cancer that can be attributed to screening. The NCI then withdrew its support of mammograms for women under 50. But the ACS refuted the study and announced it would not change its recommendation. There has been a great deal of controversy about the statistical studies that were reviewed. The medical community is faced with having to take a position even though the statistical results are inconclusive. The current question is not a statistical one; it is a political policy one. Given that we do not know whether or not mammograms save lives for women under 50, should health insurers be required to pay for them?

Certainly statistics is not a silver bullet to solve all problems. But for the physician leader, statistics can assist in the decision process of collecting, analyzing, and interpreting data. Perhaps this reminder on the desk might have value: *In God we trust; all others bring data.*

GLOSSARY

analysis of variance (ANOVA). statistical procedure of studying how the variation in a response variable is related to the levels of one or more treatment variables.

confidence interval. statement based on a sample of data that gives the interval containing the value of a population parameter. The confidence level specifies the confidence we have that the interval does include the parameter value.

correlation coefficient. numerical measure of the association between two continuous variables.

double-blind study. study in which neither the subject nor the observer knows which of several alternative treatments the subject has received. It is termed a randomized double blind if case treatment assignment is done randomly.

experimental design. assignment of specified levels of treatment variables to the units in a sample.

histogram. graph of the values of a variable plotted on the X axis versus the frequency of each value on the Y axis.

hypothesis test. statistical procedure based on sample data that chooses between two competing hypotheses termed the null hypothesis and the alternative hypothesis.

inference. process of making statements about a population based on data from one or more samples.

interaction. the fact that the average response for one treatment variable varies according to the value of one or more other treatment variables. This can be shown graphically by an interaction plot.

mean. average of a set of data. The sum of the data values divided by the number of data values.

outlier. a data value in a sample that is very different from the other values.

parameter. numerical characteristic of a population of values for a specified variable (e.g., population mean, population standard deviation).

population. the set of objects (e.g., persons) about which we wish to make a statement based on a sample of data selected from the population.

probability value or p value. probability under the assumption that the null hypothesis is true and that the test statistic exceeds the value observed for the present data.

quality management. program of process improvement that seeks to identify and eradicate special causes of variation and to reduce variability.

regression. statistical procedure of relating a response variable, Y, to one or more predictor variables by finding an equation with generally small residuals.

residual. residual analysis is used to detect outliers and models that poorly fit the sample data. residual = (observed value) − (predicted value).

response variable. the response being studied as it relates to treatments applied.

sample. the subset of the population that is selected and measured in order to make statements about the population. Samples may be selected by some random process (e.g., stratified random sample, cluster sample) or by a non-random process (e.g., quota sample, judgement sample).

scatterplot. a graph that shows the association between two continuous variables by plotting points (x, y) = (value of first variable, value of second variable).

standard deviation. a commonly used measure of spread for a continuous variable.

standard error. the standard deviation of an estimated parameter value (e.g., the standard error of the mean is a measure of the variation in a sample mean.)

statistically significant. a test of hypothesis is termed statistically significant in case the calculated probability value is less than a specified value (frequently specified to be 0.05 or 0.01).

REFERENCES

Bailar, J.C. III & Mosteller, F. (Eds.). (1992). *Medical uses of statistics* (2nd ed.), Boston: NEJM Books.

Tanur, J.M., et al (Eds.) *Statistics: A guide to the biological and health sciences.* San Francisco: Holden-Day, Inc.

Utts, J.M. (1996) *Seeing through statistics.* Belmont, CA: Wadsworth Publishing Co.

CHAPTER 14

Continuous Quality Improvement—What Every Physician Leader Needs to Know

Donald E. Lighter

TABLE OF CONTENTS

EXECUTIVE SUMMARY

Physicians today understand the characteristics of quality health care—
or do they? Every medical student has been trained to make sure that all
of the details of a patient's care are managed each day, so that they understand what quality health care entails. On the other hand, explaining the
important features of quality health care has escaped the medical profession for many years. Society has become unwilling to accept a medical license as a guarantee that a person is qualified to provide quality medical
care. The concept of value as a function of quality and cost has finally
found its way into the health care delivery system after being honed for
many years in American industry.

Physician leaders are being inundated with requests for quality improvement (QI) data and plans. The standard quality assurance paradigm
that most physicians learned over the past twenty years is not sufficient to
satisfy the need for QI. American industry is very familiar with Total
Quality Management (TQM). As a result, health care organizations are
studying and implementing Continuous Quality Improvement (CQI) projects at a rapid rate. Knowledge of TQM and CQI has become an essential
component of the physician leader's set of skills. From control charts to
group process management, physician executives must be able to bring a
quality improvement focus to the contemporary health care organization.
One of the primary goals of a physician oriented executive MBA program
is to teach physician leaders how to incorporate the quality improvement
philosophy into every aspect of an organization.

As the health care industry moves into the 21st century, physician leaders will require a growing appreciation of the demand for value in health
care services. Demonstrating value means measuring quality and cost,
and the methods of determining each of these two important parameters
consume a large portion of the education in an MBA program. Physicians
with these skills will be in extraordinary demand over the next few years,
making the time invested in attaining the MBA degree one of the best investments that a physician can make.

Few issues receive more attention in today's health care market than the
quality of care provided by the modern health care delivery system. Each
time the economic environment of health care changes, a ripple effect occurs that affects the quality of care that individual patients enjoy, as well
as the livelihood of providers. Legislators and payers have learned that financial decisions virtually always affect the quality of health care, and so

the concepts of health care finance and quality of care are inextricably linked. The recognition of the need to measure quality is only the first step toward actually ensuring that health care is accessible and appropriate (Berwick, 1989). Increasingly, physicians are expected to take the lead in defining quality of health care, and so they must have a thorough understanding of the uses of QI tools for purposes like disease management, financial planning, and quality measurement.

APPLICATION OF THE QUALITY IMPROVEMENT CYCLE TO HEALTH CARE

Most physicians recognize quality health care when they see it—or do they? For many of us steeped in the traditions of the health care system, quality health care generally translates into abundant health care. People must have rapid access to the latest technology and the most sophisticated specialty care regardless of cost. The health care delivery system evolved to provide such access, and the American public rapidly came to expect the luxury of unlimited care. As the population requiring health care grew in the 1970s and 1980s, combined with the development of more advanced diagnostic and therapeutic modalities, costs suddenly became an issue. The rise in the cost of health care far exceeded the rise in the cost of living in the United States, and those who actually assumed the brunt of those increasing costs, industry and government, rebelled at the thought that health care expenditures would consume an ever increasing percentage of the country's gross domestic product. Their reaction to this new reality has shaped health care economics in the last decade of the twentieth century.

TRENDS IN HEALTH CARE ECONOMICS

Managed care approaches to health care delivery proliferated in the 1970s and 1980s, with some areas of the country forging ahead with these concepts much more rapidly than the rest of the nation. The areas of the country that have made the most progress in applying QI to health care processes tend to be those that have the greatest managed care market penetration (Joint Commission on Accreditation of Healthcare Organizations, 1992). As managed care organizations (MCOs) mature, they find that traditional cost containment approaches, like reduced inpatient utilization, have limitations and reach a point of decreasing returns. In these markets, the next phase of managed care involves application of the same methods of QI that have been effective in other industries.

The response of the health care delivery system to these changes has been predictable. On the theory that bigger is better, large-scale consolidations have consumed huge amounts of time, effort, and capital in health care organizations. Large physician management and hospital management companies have been formed with varying success, but these new organizations have experienced significant growing pains. A number of unique contractual arrangements have wed unlikely suitors; for example, hospitals and medical groups, home care agencies, and even durable medical equipment companies. Often, these combinations languish and fail because the dominant business partner's management team has little aptitude for managing health care providers outside of their core business areas and with alien business cultures. In essence, a lack of management skill leads to failure.

CQI IN AMERICAN INDUSTRY

The era of industrialization in health care has produced unusual organizational structures, and the melding of incompatible cultures has produced an opportunity for physician leaders with the vision and ability to find commonality among all the participants and stakeholders. Physician leaders have the unique ability to lead in the health care system, because they are virtually the only participants in the system with the expert knowledge to understand health care at the patient level, as well as experience working with all of the elements of the integrated delivery system. A physician leader with an appropriate knowledge base in business administration is ideally positioned to take the reins of leadership and create an effective health care system. A physician with an understanding of quality improvement technology already understands the coming paradigm in health care when cost containment strategies have reached the pinnacle of their usefulness.

Quality improvement in manufacturing has a long history in the United States and around the world. Industry icons like W. Edwards Deming, Phillip Crosby, and J. M. Juran introduced these concepts into American industry over the past fifty years, and to a large extent, were responsible for renewing the competitiveness of American industry. QI tools help reduce problems in the production and distribution of manufactured goods, but they also have been applied to companies that supply services. These service applications have lead to the present use of QI in health care.

DEMING'S FOURTEEN QUALITY PRINCIPLES

Deming was one of the most recognized pioneers in the new age of quality improvement, and he was instrumental in bringing Japan into the international trade arena following the devastation of World War II. His insightful philosophy has become the foundation of contemporary quality improvement, and perhaps more than any other quality engineer, he shaped American industry quality practices in the last two decades of the twentieth century. Deming proposed fourteen quality principles (Deming, 1989):

1. Create constancy of purpose toward improvement of product and service, with the aim to become competitive and to stay in business, and to provide jobs.
2. Adopt the new philosophy. We are in a new economic age. Western management must awaken to the challenge, must learn their responsibilities, and take on leadership for change.
3. Cease dependence on inspection to achieve quality. Eliminate the need for inspection on a mass basis by building quality into the product in the first place.
4. End the practice of awarding business on the basis of price tag. Instead, minimize total cost. Move toward a single supplier for any one item, on a long-term relationship of loyalty and trust.
5. Improve constantly and forever the system of production and service, to improve quality and productivity, and thus constantly decrease costs.
6. Institute training on the job.
7. Institute leadership. The aim of supervision should be to help people and machines and gadgets to do a better job. Supervision of management is in need of overhaul, as well as supervision of production workers.
8. Drive out fear, so that everyone may work effectively for the company.
9. Break down barriers between departments. People in research, design, sales, and production must work as a team, to foresee problems of production and in use that may be encountered with the product or service.

10. Eliminate slogans, exhortations, and targets for the work force ask-
    ing for zero defects and new levels of productivity. Such exhorta-
    tions only create adversarial relationships, as the bulk of the causes
    of low quality and low productivity belong to the system and thus
    lie beyond the power of the work force.
    • Eliminate work standards (quotas) on the factory floor. Substi-
      tute leadership.
    • Eliminate management by objective. Eliminate management by
      numbers, numerical goals. Substitute leadership.
11. Remove barriers that rob the hourly worker of his right to pride of
    workmanship. The responsibility of supervisors must be changed
    from sheer numbers to quality.
12. Remove barriers that rob people in management and in engineering
    of their right to pride of workmanship. This means, inter alia, abol-
    ishment of the annual or merit rating and of management by objec-
    tive.
13. Institute a vigorous program of education and self-improvement.
14. Put everybody in the company to work to accomplish the transfor-
    mation. The transformation is everybody's job.

These principles led to the development of QI approaches that changed
the focus of enlightened managers from trying to change people to changing processes to improve output, and reduce cost through redesign and
reengineering. Cogent physicians have recognized these principles in
medical practice since the dawn of modern medicine. Practitioners frequently change treatment regimens to fit an individual patient's need,
while remaining within the parameters of the therapeutic modality. Fitting
the curative environment to individual variation is important to achieving
health goals, and that same approach applied to management promotes
improvements in worker productivity.

JURAN—THE FOUNDATION OF TQM

Another influential figure in twentieth century quality improvement is
J. M. Juran, whose quality trilogy codified the conceptual framework for
TQM. Briefly, the Juran paradigm entails three critical components:

• Plan
• Control
• Improve

SHEWART—THE PDSA CYCLE

Building on Walter Shewhart's Plan-Do-Study-Act cycle (Figure 14–1), Juran's comprehensive approach mandates careful planning before proceeding with any process modifications. Additionally, though, Juran extends Deming's emphasis on measurement to make it one of the defining characteristics of the TQM paradigm. Deemed "performance measures," these metrics gauge important attributes of the target process. The Agency for Health Care Policy and Research (AHCPR) used this approach when it commissioned the Institute of Medicine to formulate the concept of Clinical Practice Guidelines in 1987 (Lohr, 1992). The use of performance measures to determine the efficacy of process interventions is a key component of quality improvement in health care. In Figure 14–2, the lower cycle demonstrates the basic approach to improving a process (e.g., management of a clinical disorder) and it incorporates Shewhart's PDSA

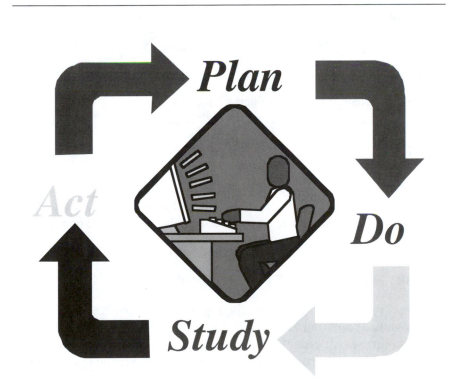

Figure 14–1 Plan-Do-Study-Act Cycle

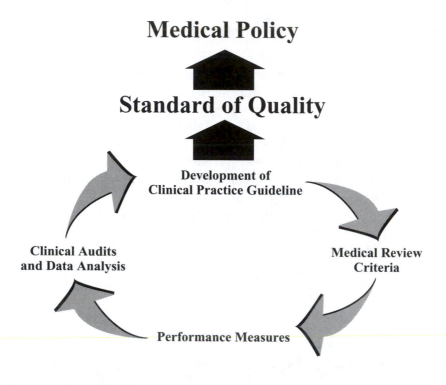

Figure 14–2 Medical Policy Development Process

model. After several iterations of the improvement cycle, standards of quality (best practices) can be inferred, and when acceptable to the medical community, these standards can be codified into medical policy. Physicians will readily recognize this approach as evidence-based medicine, which, from a scientific standpoint, has always been the goal of dedicated practitioners.

CROSBY—THE CONCEPT OF ZERO DEFECTS

Philip Crosby is credited with bringing the concept of "zero defects" to TQM (McLaughlin and Kaluzny, 1994). In manufacturing, such a goal should optimize cost reduction by reducing waste and rework, as well as increasing profits by maximizing output. In health care, such goals can be applied to performance measures like immunization rates, cervical cancer screening rates, or nosocomial infection rates. For example, when determining what mammography rates are acceptable to a provider organization, the goal should invariably be 100%, not 60% or 80%. Additionally, though, the zero defects concept applies to the final output of a process, which in the health care industry is deemed the outcome. Thus, outcome measures have become critical in determining the efficacy of a health care process, whether the process is a surgical procedure or a medical treatment regimen. Defining outcomes has become an active area of research supported by payers and government agencies, alike. Whether measures are for processes or outcomes, however, quality improvement interventions must target 100% rates, and then move inexorably toward that goal using the techniques of quality engineering. Learning approaches to leading the health care system in accomplishing such difficult objectives must be one of the primary goals of a physician leader.

QUALITY IMPROVEMENT TOOLS

Quality engineers have innumerable tools to achieve process and outcome improvement. Although these tools have been applied in industry for decades, they have only recently found champions in health care. Part of the reason for their increasing adoption by health care managers is the reliance on statistical thinking rather than rigorous statistical analysis. Most physicians remember those painful experiences with statistics on the educational road to medical practice, and many acquired a strong aversion to the rigor of statistical analysis. Statistical thinking is the approach of quality engineers that utilizes descriptive statistics to validate quality evaluations, but hides the gruesome mathematical details from analysts. Descriptive statistics includes mean, variance, and standard deviation that are very familiar to most physicians. The application of these tools to evaluation of quality improvement opportunities is the basis of quality engineering, and conceptually can be rapidly assimilated by physician leaders. Quality engineers have seven classic tools available (Mears, 1995):

- Problem identification
  1. Pareto Charts
  2. Ishikawa diagrams
  3. Histograms
  4. Run charts
- Data collection
  5. Checksheets

- Intervention design
  6. Flowcharts
- Process control
  7. Control charts

These tools have come to define the classic approach to quality improvement, and they are used to insure that each step in the PDSA cycle provides valid conclusions. Problem identification tools define the source of variation in a process, allowing planning to decrease inappropriate variation and improve quality. Exhibit 14–1 provides examples of these four tools. In order to validate the problems identified, data must be collected and analyzed, and checksheet (data collection sheet) design provides a scientific approach to gathering information to improve the validity of decisions and interventions.

Flow Charts

Flowcharting has proven extremely valuable for health care managers in understanding and optimizing processes. Often, the very act of producing a flowchart uncovers problems in process flow that respond to simple intervention (Cordes, 1998). In more complex processes, flowcharting may present the only means of understanding the true structure of a system. Variations of flowcharting (e.g., PERT charts) provide a means of capturing the sequence of resource utilization to promote "just in time" inventory systems that reduce cost and waste. Figure 14–3 presents a flow chart that was created for the diagnosis of asthma in children.

Control Charts

Finally, control charts have become the classic tools of Statistical Process Control (SPC) in American industry (Wise and Fair, 1998). Control charts typically chart lines for the mean and three standard deviations above and below the mean, over which data collection points are plotted. Based on the patterns of data points, variations in the process that are outside expected limits can be identified and targeted for intervention. Control charts are most useful for ongoing processes in which variation is a source of cost and diminished productivity, and these statistical models allow rapid analysis and intervention for active processes. In health care, control charts are useful for analyzing performance and outcome mea-

Exhibit 14–1 Problem Identification Tools

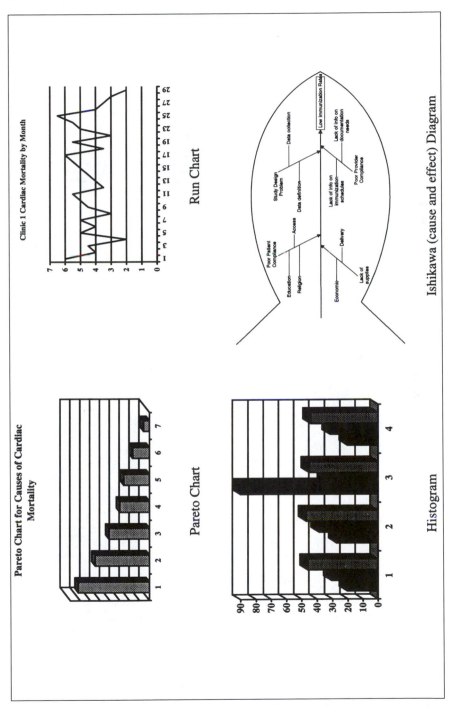

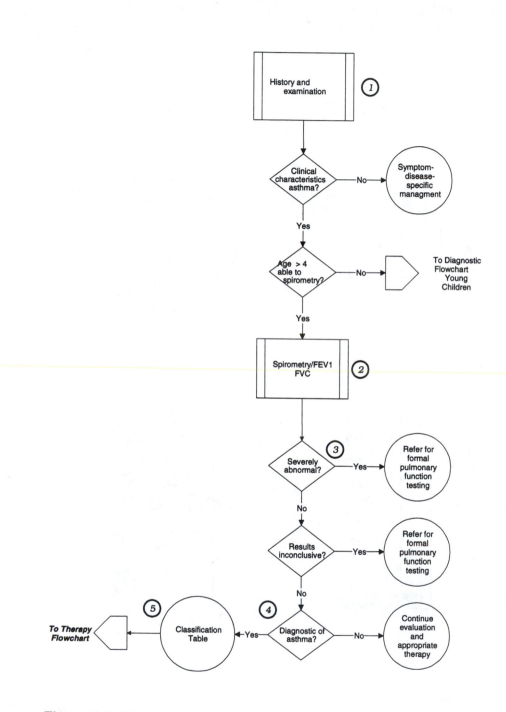

Figure 14–3 Diagnostic Flowchart for Asthma in Children

sures in diagnostic and therapeutic systems of care for specific disorders or preventive care. Using control charts, health care managers can usually identify sources of variation that determine approaches for improvement. Figure 14–4 demonstrates a control chart for waiting times for an outpatient clinic. Upper and lower control limits are set at ± 3 standard deviations from the mean so that "out of control" points may be identified easily. An out of control process is one in which special effects (termed special causes in SPC) create problems for providing products or services using the current process. Control charts make identification of problem areas much more precise, and over the next few years in health care, these tools will become increasingly important.

GOALS OF TQM AND CQI

One of the advantages of the TQM approach in health care is the introduction of an evidence-based approach to decision making. One of the major criticisms of managed health care in the United States is the lack of a scientific basis for the recommendations for care made by managed care

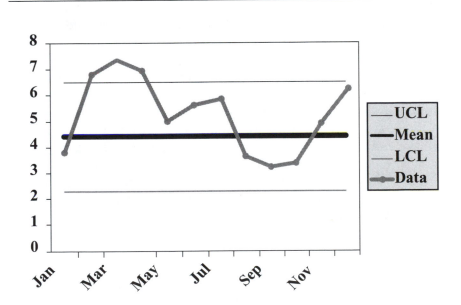

Figure 14–4 Control Chart for Waiting Times in the Outpatient Clinic

medical directors (Abelson, 1998; Jeffrey, 1998). Since a substantial majority of medical care is based on an individual clinician's experience, rather than scientific evidence, many decisions on medical necessity lack the kind of scientific validity that physicians desire. Thus, disputes arise due to disagreements on the meaning of disparate clinical experience. TQM proposes to gradually add scientific and statistical validity to the decision making process by using the wealth of clinical and administrative data accumulating in the health care industry to define efficacious practice patterns. Additionally, the TQM approach insures that the analysis continues indefinitely as medical science advances and improves the effectiveness of clinical medicine. The utility of data in the CQI process should be intuitively evident; in fact, the central dogma in CQI can be stated, "In God we trust, all others bring data."

CONCLUSION

In summary, then, the study of CQI and TQM is crucial for physician leaders to effectively promote cost effective, high quality health care. Payers are demanding data on the quality of services to determine the value of those services, and they also expect health care systems to implement improvement programs, just as they have over the past several decades. The need to improve patient care and contain costs will become more important as the global economy demands increased competitiveness, and so payers will no longer tolerate breaches in quality of care as reimbursement declines. Although difficult to discern in the current environment of medical economics, the switch to a quality improvement paradigm will also improve physicians' satisfaction with medical practice, as the focus of their work will return to providing quality health care to patients (Foulke et. al., 1998). By emphasizing the customer (patient) in the health care delivery system, advanced diagnostic and therapeutic interventions will be created that help physicians in the next century gain increased satisfaction with the work performed on behalf of the central figures in the health care system—patients.

GLOSSARY

checksheets. data collection sheets designed to eliminate errors and improve efficiency of data collection.

clinical practice guideline. systematically developed statements to assist practitioners' and patients' decisions about health care to be provided for specific clinical circumstances.

continuous quality improvement (CQI). the philosophy espoused by Deming, Juran, Crosby, and others of perpetually trying to enhance the quality of products or services that are the product of an organization's business efforts.

control chart. a chart of a parameter of interest; for example, a performance measure, over time, including upper and lower control limits to determine the stability of a process over time.

CQI. continuous quality improvement.

evidence-based medicine. medical care based on scientific evidence obtained from published medical literature sources or from consensus panels of experts.

flow chart. a graphical representation of a process.

Ishikawa diagram. also known as a Fishbone diagram; a graphical representation of relationships between causes and effects of a quality problem, allowing grouping of root causes.

managed care organizations (MCOs). organizations (e.g., health maintenance organizations and some preferred provider organizations) that contract with payers to supervise patient care in a population.

Pareto chart. a histogram of data arranged in order of descending data values; based on the Pareto Rule (the 80–20 rule) that 80% of the errors in a process emanate from 20% of the process components.

PDSA. Plan-Do-Study-Act.

performance measures. parameters measured as a result of studying a process that gauges the ability of the process to achieve its goal in terms of quality and output.

PERT chart. Program Evaluation and Review Technique Chart; variant of flow chart.

Plan-Do-Study-Act cycle. originally proposed by Walter Shewhart, the PDSA cycle is the methodologic approach to quality improvement activities in which a process is studied for designing a plan for intervention, the intervention is implemented, and the effects of the implementation are studied, followed by action to improve the process. The cycle is repeated until process quality has been optimized.

QI. quality improvement.

quality engineer. a professional trained in the techniques of quality improvement and TQM.

quality improvement cycle. the steps necessary to perform quality improvement analyses and interventions.

run chart. a graphical depiction of data points over time with specific analytic implications in determining the types of causes of quality problems.

statistical thinking. the process of evaluating a process using simple descriptive statistics to better understand the nature of problems embedded in the system.

Total Quality Management (TQM). a management philosophy that promotes the permeation of quality improvement techniques and interventions throughout the entire organization.

REFERENCES

Berwick, D. (1989). Continuous improvement as an ideal in health care. *New England Journal of Medicine, 320,* 53–56.

Cordes, R.M. (1998). Flowcharting: An essential tool. *Quality Digest, 6,* 31–34.

Deming, W.E. (1986). *Out of the crisis.* Cambridge MA: Massachusetts Institute of Technology, Center for Advanced Engineering Study.

Foulke, G.E., Bell, R.A., Siefkin, A.D., Kravitz, R.L. (1998). Attitudes and behavioral intentions regarding managed care: A comparison of academic and community physicians. *American Journal of Managed Care, 4,* 555–563.

Jeffrey, N.A. (1998). Doctor discipline boards are seen as new threat for HMOs. *Wall Street Journal,* p. 1.

Joint Commission on Accreditation of Healthcare Organizations. (1992). *Striving for improvement: Six hospitals in search of quality.* Oakbrook Terrace, IL: Author.

Lohr, K.N. (1992). Reasonable expectations: From the Institute of Medicine [interview by Paul M. Schyve]. *QRB Quality Review Bulletin, 18,* 393–396.

McLaughlin, C., & Kaluzny, A. (1994). *Continuous quality improvement in health care: Theory, implementation, and applications.* Gaithersburg, MD: Aspen Publishers.

Mears, P. (1995). *Quality improvement tools and techniques.* New York: McGraw-Hill.

Wise, S., & Fair, D. (1998). *Innovative control charting: practical spc solutions for today's manufacturing environment.* Milwaukee, WI: ASQ Quality Press.

CHAPTER 15

Diagnosing the Security of Your Organization's Information

Amy W. Ray

TABLE OF CONTENTS

EXECUTIVE SUMMARY

Information networks have become the lifeblood of nearly every type of business in the world. Vendors and customers used to be surprised and delighted with immediate responsiveness to special requests. Now they demand it. Building and maintaining highly effective information networks is critically important to providing the kind of responsiveness demanded today.

The health care field faces special challenges as administrators and providers work with technology experts to develop integrated patient records that seamlessly interface with business information systems. As the integration between clinical systems and business systems within local health care systems improves, the ability to share information across geographically dispersed health care systems will also improve. Eventually, physicians from different countries will immediately and reliably be able to view the same patient record.

Unfortunately, increased connectivity also means increased vulnerability. Creating external connections to internal information makes information more accessible to unauthorized as well as authorized users of information. Information security is doubly important in health care because patient records as well as financial information must be protected. The purpose of this chapter is to provide a high level overview of primary risks and corresponding measures of protection that health care business leaders should take to reduce risk of lost, stolen, or corrupted data in a connected environment.

REWARDS AND RISKS OF SHARING INFORMATION

We are living in a wired world. If big news breaks, the media immediately and explicitly shares every fact and potential fact they can get their hands on. The same networks and satellites that send information to news reporters also transfer valuable business information to firms around the globe. The executive managers of leading businesses know that being immediately responsive to vendors and customers is critically important and there is a positive correlation between connectivity and firm responsiveness. Unfortunately, increased connectivity also means increased vulnerability. The purpose of this chapter is to provide a high level overview of primary risks and measures of protection that firm managers should take to reduce risk of lost, stolen, or corrupted data in a connected environment.

Connecting Internal Systems

Virtually every industry is challenged to creatively exploit advances in information technology. New information sources are constantly emerging and the reasons and methods for sharing information are limited only by our imaginations. The health care field faces special challenges as administrators and providers work with technology experts to develop integrated patient records that seamlessly interface with business information systems. The large transaction volume in most health care information systems adds to the challenge of maintaining the integrity of data captured in those systems. For example, in most health care information systems the following is possible:

- information regarding one patient resides in many different files.
- several users may attempt to access or update a single file at the same time.
- each user may have access to multiple databases.

Without proper security and controls, this environment is ripe for recording errors. Another complication is the fact that a hospital may have thousands of types of just one supply item, such as sutures. Families of supplies are usually numbered similarly so update errors in a family of supplies with a thousand members are likely to occur unless the appropriate management policies and recording techniques are used. Information security, as it is practiced in such mundane activities as ensuring sutures are recorded properly, is every bit as important to the financial health of an organization as the information security applied to keeping out the riff-raff.

In large health care networks, multiple names and codes for the same procedure may exist. When Kaiser Permanente decided to standardize its information coding scheme, it found that there were as many as nine codes for one surgical procedure. Health care administrators are continuously faced with increasing demands on their abilities to improve communication, collaboration, and coordination, of efforts through the more effective use of their information networks.

Connecting to the World

Although much emphasis is currently placed on improving internal networks in nearly every industry, perhaps even more effort is exerted in leading firms to establish superior networks with strategic business partners. Many health care organizations are also working to provide public service information networks, develop integrated delivery systems, implement enterprise-wide information systems, or complete countless other networking projects. After exerting all the effort required to simply get connected, who has the time, energy, or money to implement and monitor the security of those systems and networks? Ironically, without the additional effort to secure connections properly, those connections can invite financial disaster into an organization.

Security is especially important for organizations with Internet connections. The advantage of using the Internet is that it is public, so it is free. The disadvantage to using the Internet is that it is public, so with the aid of some inexpensive and readily available software, virtually anyone can read data you transmit over the Internet. However, there are ways to use the Internet that decrease an organization's risk dramatically. For example, when two firms decide to set up a dedicated line of communication for information exchange, there are several options available. The most expensive is to put in place a complete, private network. A rather inexpensive option that many firms are choosing today is to implement a virtual private network (VPN). VPNs may include many bells and whistles but are primarily communications over the Internet that are encrypted with proprietary algorithms shared only by the engaging firms. Further discussion on secure use of the Internet could fill a book and is beyond the scope of this chapter. If you are considering such actions, please engage a consultant or other expert.

KNOW THE ENEMIES

There are several categories of people that pose a security threat to an organization's information system. The major categories that every administrator should consider are discussed here in order from the most exciting to read about to the least, which is coincidentally also the order of least important to most.

Competitive Spies and Teenagers

When you start to think about who might pose a security threat to your information networks, the mind cannot help but wander to thoughts of cunning and sinister villains from novels you would take to the beach. Either the villain is destroying computer networks in an attempt to achieve world dominance or the villain has a personal axe to grind with the hero. Seriously, industrial espionage is in fact sharply on the rise, in part due to the world's increasing connectivity. Company documents, computer aided designs (CAD), and marketing plans are particularly valued items to steal electronically (Davis, 1997). However, while industrial espionage exists, computer crimes committed by employees inside an organization represent five times the number of crimes committed by competitors (five times!) (Smith, 1998). Accidental data losses resulting from poor data management are more than twice the data losses from all categories of intentional fraud put together. Ensuring proper management and security of data inside the firm's walls should be the primary focus of any company's plan.

Before moving on, it is worth mentioning another category of external threat: teenagers and hackers. A hacker is a person who illegally gains access to and sometimes tampers with information in a computer system. Studies on hackers indicate that on average hackers are young, they do not have full-time jobs nor do they own property (Winkler, 1998). That profile sounds a lot like a teenager. An FBI agent with twenty years of experience in solving computer crimes told this author that teenagers scare him much more than older, experienced criminals. This is not to say that teenagers are inherently bad, but a teenager that becomes obsessed with the Internet may potentially start hanging out with strange cyber-fellows. Armed with large amounts of time, extraordinary comfort with computers and no apparent understanding of the consequences suffered by the real people that depend on those computers, breaking through corporate firewalls simply becomes a test of skill. Virtual gangs have emerged on the Internet that have contests to see who can break into Company X's network first. Incidentally, the emergence of VPNs and related technologies may have the effect of simply making the contest more 'fun'. Again, such threats should not be the primary focus of an organization's security plan, but if there are strong basic managerial and technological defenses in place, efforts to recognize symptoms of such attacks and act expediently are worth the additional investment. Remember—you may be paranoid, but they still may be out to get you.

Information Week and Ernst & Young conduct an annual information security survey. Respondents include information system chiefs, information security officers, and other high ranking information technology personnel. One trend in the survey results from year to year is the increasing paranoia about outsiders. Out of 627 respondents from the United States in 1997, 75% believe that authorized users of company systems pose a security threat, 70% see computer terrorists as a threat, and 42% see competitors as a threat. Interestingly, 61% also see consultants and auditors as a threat.

Yet in the midst of all this paranoia, it is also interesting to note that 82% of companies in the United States link their corporate networks to the Internet, and a whopping 22% say they are moving vital data via the Internet. These statistics are slightly higher than the collective worldwide statistics. Internationally, 70% of firms have Internet connections and 10% have vital information on the Internet. At least for the time being, it appears that the general belief is that external connections provide added value above and beyond the associated risks.

The Quiet Ones

The overwhelming majority of attacks on information networks come from insiders. Studies of computer criminals have revealed recognizable patterns of behavior during the period when the crime takes place as well as patterns of behavior in their personal lives that managers may use to recognize potential problems.

Stealing from a company is easiest when collusion is involved. When two employees with complementary job responsibilities decide to work together to pull off a theft, it is pretty hard to catch them. Fortunately, most thieves are either too cowardly or too greedy to involve others in their plans. When one employee acts alone, managerial controls should be in place that facilitate identification of unusual activities. For example, if a clerk records a withdrawal of cash there must be some related activity such as an increase in supplies. Small thefts are harder to catch than big ones, so a smart thief may repetitively steal smaller quantities. This type of thief is the most common and is also the type that usually starts behaving differently after a while. The following are new behaviors that may signal a problem:

- The employee becomes highly protective of his or her own work.
- The employee exhibits new nervous habits such as reduced eye contact or shortness of temper.
- The employee may become unwilling or reluctant to take vacations or time off.

A survey of people convicted of stealing from their employers revealed some additional surprising facts (Romney, Steinbart, & Cushing, 1997). The majority of respondents fit the following description:

- The individual had access to the information used to commit the crime long before the crime was committed.
- The individual noted that he or she were only borrowing from the company and intended to return everything at a later date.
- Nearly every individual mentioned that a personal financial crisis had occurred prior to the act. Noted crises include everything from caring for a critically ill child to maintaining a personal drug habit or gambling debt.

It is interesting to note that absent from the list are the disgruntled employees that are taking revenge on the company. There may be a couple of reasons why there are not as many recorded cases of this category of theft. Perhaps most likely, it is embarrassing to an organization's management if they do not see a predictable attack coming that leaves the company in a vulnerable position. Management may strike a deal with the offender that does not involve prosecution so that no official record is established. Studies indicate that only about 10% of the identified attacks against computer systems are ever actually reported (Kabay, 1998). Another reason why vengeance probably did not make it into the incarcerated's top ten list of 'Why I Did It' is that such admissions probably would not sit very well with a parole board.

The Sly Ones

Sometimes confidential information is obtained by piecing together small bits of information. This is referred to as leakage by inference. A large number of personnel may have access to a patient's record. However, each person should only have access to the portion of the record needed to complete his or her tasks. Creating such controls is one of the primary responsibilities of database managers in companies with strong information systems. The information management personnel create individual 'views' for each type of database user. Well-designed views only allow users access to the information needed in order to perform their jobs. Therefore, employees performing financial tasks should only have views to pertinent financial information. Employees performing health care tasks on the other hand should only have access to pertinent health care information. An added benefit to having well-designed views is that they actually make tasks easier for employees to complete by eliminating excess clutter from the screen.

In many health care settings, especially smaller ones, paper documents are still used and either separation of duties is performed manually or the staff is smaller and highly trusted. However, as electronic patient records grow in use and centers of care grow in size, it is important to consider electronic separation of duties more carefully. Reasons for providing this sort of control run the gamut from protecting the confidentiality of patients to protecting confidential organizational financial and other information from busybodies.

The Unwitting Ones

It is important to educate handlers of confidential information to ensure that they realize the seriousness of maintaining confidentiality. Policies and procedures should be established and strictly enforced for protecting sensitive data. Everyone from executive management to volunteers should go through basic training concerning the maintenance of patient confidentiality. Even employees with good intentions may accidentally leave confidential patient records in a vulnerable state. For example, one important managerial policy is to ensure that all patient files, physical and electronic, are secure when employees leave the site of use.

With all the frenetic activity in a normal health care setting it is easy to relax enforcement of such policies. However lack of adherence can be very costly to the organization and may include everything from loss of data to lawsuits from patients to complete loss of markets. There are stories of blatant recklessness with patient confidentiality, which exemplify the latter extreme. In February 1997, a hospital in Sheffield, England needed a little help with its data processing, so it literally started grabbing people off the street and set them to processing over 50,000 confidential gynecological records.

To ensure that all handlers of confidential information understand the importance of discretion, all employees should be required to go through sensitivity and confidentiality training and be required to sign legally binding confidentiality and nondisclosure agreements. In addition, patients should be educated about their rights to fair treatment and confidentiality. Such practices not only protect the patients, but also the physicians by ensuring that everyone knows how information is and should be used throughout the system.

AN OUNCE OF PREVENTION . . .

Every information security plan should include elements of prevention and detection. Of course preventing security breeches is far preferred to detecting them. Therefore, the focus of the remainder of this chapter is going to be on effective preventive measures in a company's security defense plan. Specifically, authentication and encryption techniques, physical security of equipment, prevention and detection of viruses, disaster recovery, and most importantly, managerial policies will be covered.

There are no guarantees that network security will not be breached. However, remembering three simple guidelines can be very useful in strengthening organizational defenses:

1. Information security is provided in layers and the more layers an organization has, the better it will be protected
2. No matter how technologically advanced the defense mechanisms are, they will not be effective without managerial enforcement of their proper use.
3. Triage is the best approach to implementing security measures. Identify mission critical systems and secure those first. Beyond mission critical systems, it is a good idea to ensure internal security and to limit external connections until it is viable to maintain external connections securely. The good news is that most of the measures taken to secure a network against threats from insiders help protect against threats from outsiders, although protection against outsiders does require some additional effort.

THE ACHES AND PAINS OF COMPUTER VIRUSES

The American Institute of Certified Public Accountants has started a series of books addressing computer and networking concerns facing accountants and their clients. In the book of Top Ten concerns for 1998 (Smith, 1998), the number one concern was information security. The number one information security concern was viruses. Almost every organization has had at least one computer infected with a computer virus. What viruses are and what can be done to prevent infection are discussed below.

What Viruses Are

Unfortunately, it doesn't take a genius to write a malicious computer program. Some malicious programs are written with intent to harm but most of them are actually written for sport or intellectual challenge. Like most computer-ese, the term virus is used loosely in reference to many nasty things that are not really viruses. All garden-variety types of malicious code, including worms and trojan horses and even non-malicious but problematic code such as the year 2000 problem, are often referred to as viruses. However, a virus has two distinct characteristics:

- A virus must be attached to executable code.
- A virus is designed to copy itself into other files.

How prolific a virus becomes depends upon how well written it is and how often the associated executable code is called. Viruses are one of the favorite playthings of beginning hacker "wannabes." Unfortunately, there are actually build-your-own virus toolkits on the market that make it easy for those wannabes to get started. Anti-virus software continues to become more sophisticated as well, but it's not likely that the gaming will end anytime soon. Ironically, the user-friendliness and sophistication of our most standard business software also has a role in the proliferation of viruses. Just a few years ago, the world took comfort in the fact that viruses couldn't be attached to a simple data file. However, word processors have become quite sophisticated and while simple data files still don't pass along viruses, word processor generated templates that contain macros, or small bits of executable code, can pass along viruses. What all this means is that there are no bulletproof solutions. However, the more precautions that management takes, the lower the risk of data loss. Some helpful management policies include the following:

- No software should be downloaded over the organization's network from the Internet.
- All new or nonstandard software should be scanned with anti-virus software and checked by information services before it is loaded on an employee's computer.
- Disks should be scanned with anti-virus software before each use.

The Frustrating Surprises

The International Computer Security Association notes that at last count there were over 8,000 identifiable viruses collectively detectable through use of anti-virus software (Kabay, 1998). The real kicker is that out of all those viruses, only 2% are inherently damaging or capable of destroying data. Yet all viruses result in lost time and money. It takes time to eradicate viruses and before even harmless viruses are detected they may significantly degrade system performance by noticeably slowing system response times. In worst cases, degradation may be significant enough to crash the system.

HOW DO I KNOW YOU'RE YOU?

User authentication is critically important to the security of a firm's information systems because it is the first preventative measure that a firm can take against lost, stolen, or corrupted data. Available authentication techniques range in sophistication from passwords and physical identification cards to digital signatures, digital certificates, and biometric measures to prevent unauthorized users from entering the system. It doesn't take a rocket scientist to figure out that highly confidential information merits the use of more highly sophisticated authentication procedures while general control over network access may be accomplished adequately through simpler techniques. It is important to note that the purpose of authentication procedures is to ensure accountability for use of information. Passwords and identification cards, the two most widely accepted authentication techniques, can be transferred to other users. Therefore it is critically important that managerial policies addressing protection and control of authentication methods be strictly enforced.

Passwords

The most commonly known and widely used form of authentication is the password. In fact, nearly 80% of businesses use passwords as their primary means of security (*Network Authentication Solutions,* 1997). Passwords are easy to implement, inexpensive to maintain, and can be used in a variety of ways. For example, one password may allow a user to log into a system while another password may be required to secure access to a confidential file requested by a user. Passwords can also be used by database administrators as a means for limiting access to user views. In the case of the financial clerk discussed earlier, when the clerk enters a password it should be automatically matched with an information access table to control the user's view.

Passwords should be changed frequently, should not be written down anywhere and should be easy for the user to remember but difficult for someone else to figure out.

This author once had a student tell about his roommate's adventures during a part-time job at a large bank. The roommate happened upon a list of users just lying on a co-workers desk. For some reason, this was enough to inspire him to play games that eventually cost him his internship.

From the list, he quickly wrote down the user identification (ID) of one of the bank's vice presidents (VP). The next day the student called the VP's wife and told her that he was a reporter for the local newspaper and that he wanted to feature a story on her highly successful husband. Flattered, she quickly agreed and he began a series of questions: what is your name, do you have any children, what are their names, do you have any pets, what are their names. After the mock interview, the student attempted to log onto the bank's computers from his home using the VP's ID. Armed with the news bits so willingly supplied by the VP's spouse, through trial and error the student finally discovered that the VP's password was the dog's name. Supposedly, he had no malicious intent, he just wanted to see if he could get in. While he was apparently clever enough to figure out what the VP's password was, he was not clever enough to figure out that the bank's computer logs would flag the unusual activity and trace the log on point to the student's computer. The punchline is the best part. The student's punishment was to give a presentation to the bank board explaining what he had done, how he had done it, and how the bank could prevent it from ever happening again. What is the moral of the story? Don't ever leave system access information such as user IDs lying around in any accessible form. Another secondary moral is that while passwords should be easy to remember, they should not be easy to figure out. The best defense is to have a policy that users should combine some series of meaningful numbers and characters. Many computer systems are configured so that known proper nouns and words found in the dictionary will not be accepted by the system as valid passwords.

A final word on the use of passwords in a health care environment. On average, logging on to a system requires approximately 30 seconds. While this is acceptable in the business office, 30 seconds may be an eternity in an operating room. Special biometric authentication methods are evolving specifically for such settings and are discussed in the biometrics section below.

Physical Identification Cards

Physical identification cards are tokens that are required of the user for authentication. Tokens may be used alone or in combination with additional knowledge that the user possesses. They may be as simple as electronic badges used for gaining access to a room, building, or piece of equipment or they can be smart cards which carry microprocessors that can exchange information with a system to provide even higher levels of security.

The advantages and disadvantages of tokens and passwords are similar. For both of these authentication procedures, the system grants access to the item, not the person. If an intruder guesses a password or finds a token, the system will allow the intruder to enter. A unique problem with simple tokens is that they are easy to forge. For that reason, tokens are often used in combination with passwords. An ATM card is an excellent example of this.

Encryption

Everyone at one time or another has tried to decode the crypto-quotes in the daily newspaper. These brainteasers use simple substitution encryption techniques where one letter is substituted for another and once the pattern is discovered then the message can be decoded. Such encryption techniques date back at least to Caesar. Encryption techniques used for transferring information across networks today are far more sophisticated. So sophisticated in some cases that the United States government would like to prevent them from being use internationally. The theory is that if messages are so strongly encrypted that they cannot be cracked by national security, what is to prevent terrorists from using these techniques to freely conduct business or steal important secrets? This is a valid point. On the other side of the fence are business managers in the United States feeling as though they are missing out on a lot of business opportunities with all the other countries that use strong encryption techniques. This too is a valid point, and it is unclear exactly who will win this argument.

According to Jim Heath of Viacorp (Heath, 1997–1998), there are four main reasons why use of strong encryption will continue to grow in the business community:

1. Computers are everywhere and connections are highly decentralized. When businesses were all hierarchically designed and infor-

mation systems were centralized, information never left the internal network, so encryption was not that important. Today, having point of entry controls are not enough. Information needs to be protected as it is en route and the best way to do that is through message encryption.

2. Information travels along unsecured networks such as the Internet making it highly vulnerable to snoopers.

3. Faxes are vulnerable to electronic and physical message interception and are not a solution to the confidentiality problem

4. Since 1977, we have had publicly available encryption techniques which solve many of the problems of the old symmetric cyphers and make transmission of encrypted messages much more convenient. These systems are called public key algorithms, and a method called RSA was the first to become commercially successful. Public key algorithms actually require two keys to function, one public and one private.

You cannot do the math in your head for public key encryption, so don't try. Just trust that it works like this:

*   Each person has his or her own private key and public key.
*   The public key for person A is published and is readily available to anyone that wants to send a message to person A.
*   When person B wants to send a message to A, B composes the message then encrypts it with A's public key and then sends the encrypted message to A.

Once the message reaches A, A must use the private key to decrypt the message. In other words, the keys work together to unlock the message and only the holder of the private key can do that. Public key encryption techniques are also referred to as asymmetric encryption techniques since two different keys are required to unlock the message.

Digital Signatures

The growth in popularity of public key encryption techniques for sending information across networks has led to some innovative new ideas for user authentication. If a user already has a private key, then he or she already possesses an encryption algorithm that is uniquely his or hers. This unique algorithm may then be used to create an electronic 'signature' for that individual. In this way, the intended recipient has assurance that the message did in fact come from the trusted sender and that the message has not been altered during its transmission.

As an example, a physician could send information to a pharmacist regarding prescription information for a patient. If the physician and the pharmacist already have a trusted electronic relationship then the pharmacist has a copy of the physician's public key. This provides the pharmacist with assurance that the message is not coming from someone pretending to be the physician. In other words, if an intruder posed as the physician and encrypted a message with a counterfeit private key, the actual physician's public key would not decode the message and the pharmacist would know that the message was fraudulent. In this way, the process of encrypting a message creates a digital signature.

In practice, the mathematical complexities of strong asymmetric encryption techniques consume large sums of computational resources and are therefore impractical as a means of encrypting all electronic transmissions. An alternative to strongly encrypting an entire message is to create a digest of the original message text. For example, every 21st character of the message could be selected and used to create a string of characters now known as the message digest. By applying the private key algorithm to the message digest, authentication can still take place. While this method does not prevent an intruder from reading the text of the message, it does prevent the intruder from changing the text of the message, because the message digest must still match the message sent. This technique represents a trade-off of transmission efficiency for complete message privacy. Yet another possibility is to use a private key for creating a digital signature and a symmetric algorithm such as the substitution algorithm discussed earlier for encrypting the text since symmetric algorithms take up far fewer resources. Business guidelines for appropriate use of various techniques need to be established within a firm.

Digital Certificates

While digital signatures have come into existence as a result of public key encryption techniques, digital certificates represent an outgrowth of the digital signature technology. Fortunately, learning how digital certificates work is much easier than learning how digital signatures work. Digital signatures work great as long as a company only does business with other companies with whom they have working, trusted relationships. However, what if a health care clinic in another country sends you a message requesting information that you would not mind sharing with a real health clinic but you would mind sharing with a hacker? Even if the senders are legitimate and use a digital signature, since you have never done business with them before you have no way of knowing if the persons are who they say they are.

This is where digital certificates come in. Anyone who uses public key encryption can have his or her keys registered with a third party, who is in turn responsible for authentication of either or both parties. So the next question is, 'How do you know you can trust the third party?' As use of this business practice grows, organizations such as Visa, MasterCard, and the U.S. Postal Service are vying to be trusted third-party authenticators. It is the combined use of digital signatures, digital certificates, and various forms of encryption that is enabling secure global electronic commerce.

Biometrics

Biometric measures, such as facial maps, retinal scans, iris scans, hand geometry recognition, fingerprints, and voice prints, are being used more frequently for identification purposes. Biometrics is considered to be more secure than passwords or smart cards since biometrics represent something that you are, not something that you possess. You may forget to bring along your smart card or you may forget what your password is, but it's pretty hard to forget to bring along a part of your body.

Another reason why biometric measures are gaining favor with the medical community is that they generally require less time and less fuss when logging on to a system. They do however require the installation of additional expensive peripheral equipment for reading the chosen body part. Viable biometrics touted in various research studies include facial maps, retinal scans, iris scans, hand geometry recognition, finger prints, and voice prints. Readers or scanners for most of these biometrics are fairly robust. Once the mechanisms have been installed to compare live with recorded samples, no additional equipment is necessary.

A great deal of research has been done with voice recognition systems in the medical community as a means of capturing and maintaining patient information. While use of voice recognition for this purpose is still under development, use of voice recognition for user authentication is more advanced. Since voices are unique, hackers may be deterred by the possibility of having their own unique voice recorded by the security system. As with all security measures, this authentication technique is even more powerful when combined with other authentication methods such as passwords.

Facial recognition is another biometric measure that has been touted as an efficient method of authentication in the medical community. Small cameras are placed in enclosures with two-way mirrors that are placed at workstations. When the user simply looks at the mirror, the camera is used to analyze the face and match special parameters of the face with stored and encrypted data about the authorized user. When another authorized user looks into the mirror, he or she is then seamlessly authenticated. Most of these systems will lock down after the user walks away from the system.

In the event of medical emergencies, there is a dual edged information problem. Immediate access to information is essential but the information needed, for example patient medical history or lab results, should be held highly confidential. Complicating matters further, since the medical staff uses the information systems sporadically and quickly as a source of reference, and since there is usually a premium on space, several individuals may share one computer. This high level of rotation means that every time another person uses the system, he or she has to be authenticated again. Methods such as the facial recognition system described above may provide some powerful solutions to the medical community.

WHEN TO QUARANTINE YOUR COMPUTERS

Even after implementing technically advanced security measures such as facial scanners, it's critically important to remember to lock the door! Physical security should be in place to provide protection for buildings, computers, software, documents, and access tools. It is also very important to create backups of data, to have hot sites available in case of emergency, and to conducts test drills and audits to ensure that those security measures can be relied upon when necessary.

DISASTER RECOVERY

Of course, no one wants to contemplate the occurrence of a disaster, but sticking your head in the sand does little to protect you in the case of either man-made or natural disasters. It is important to have plans in place to protect your information. First and foremost, backup copies of data are absolutely essential. The old technique of maintaining three copies of all data is still quite effective. There should be a master file and two other copies each secured in different physical locations and preferably in fire-proof safes. The number of times that backups are created is dependent upon the nature of the data and the frequency of transaction processing. Large hospitals with online real-time processing may require several backups daily. For smaller organizations such as specialized clinics, daily backups at the close of business may be sufficient.

One important point to bear in mind is that in a client-server environment, data files stored on the hard drive of individual computers are not systematically backed up when files on the server are. Therefore, local data backups are the responsibility of the individuals using the computers.

Some other common sense protection measures include:

- Maintain an uninterruptable power supply.
- Take out appropriate business insurance.
- Maintain a site for continuity of service in case of disaster.

PUT IT ON PAPER

There is no doubt that in our highly connected world, sophisticated technology plays a very important role in the provision of security to our information systems. However, without strictly enforced policies and procedures to guide the use of that technology, management may only be getting a false sense of security from its investments. Policies must be well planned, carefully articulated, and distributed to all users as soon as they begin working for the firm. Some of the primary issues that should be covered in security policy statements include the following:

- a list of job descriptions along with related access authorization
- security responsibilities by job description
- security responsibilities for all employees
- clearly articulated penalties for intentional breach of security
- clearly articulated penalties for leaving access to the information system open
- procedures for physically securing equipment
- procedures for physically securing hard copies of documents
- clearly articulated nondisclosure information

- frequent security and privacy awareness programs for employees as well as patients.

GLOSSARY

biometrics. the use of human physical attributes for the purpose of electronic identification. Forms of biometrics include voice recognition, facial maps, retinal scans, iris scans, hand geometry recognition, and finger prints.

collusion. the act of two or more people working together to commit fraud.

computer virus. code segment, often malicious, that is designed to copy itself into other files and is attached to another executable file.

digital certificate. a document verifying that a public key is bound to an individual sending a message.

digital signature. authentication technique involving the use of unique algorithms in combination with electronic message text to uniquely identify the sender of the message. The purpose of a digital signature is to provide assurance to the readers of the messages that the senders are in fact who they say they are.

encryption. procedures used to convert plain text data into ciphertext in order to prevent unauthorized readers from understanding the contents of the message.

firewall. hardware, software, or a combination of both dedicated to monitoring all communications to and from outside networks. There are several firewall techniques available for monitoring and filtering information at a private network gateway.

hacker. a person who illegally gains access to and sometimes tampers with information in a computer system.

malicious code. computer program or segment of a program written with the intention of creating problems for the user of that program, including everything from simple inconveniences to complete destruction of computer files.

mission critical systems. those applications that are critical to the viability of a company. For example, accounts receivables and accounts payables are mission critical data files in all organizations.

network. the hardware, software, and communications devices that provide connectivity among computers.

password. a character string used to authenticate a user during log–on procedures.

private key. the encryption algorithm in a public key encryption scheme that is kept secret for a particular person. The private key is used to decrypt messages sent to that person that have been encrypted with the recipient's public key. It is also used to encrypt messages sent to others.

private network. an external network built and used for specific purposes. A geographically dispersed company may invest in a private network for communication among multiple sites or a vendor and large customer may use a private network for information sharing. Private networks are expensive but provide high levels of security.

public key. the encryption algorithm in a public key encryption scheme that is published for a particular person. Individuals wishing to send encrypted messages to that person use the public key to encrypt a message before sending it. Only the private key for the intended message recipient can decrypt the message.

public key encryption. an authentication technique where each person receives a public key that is published and a private key that is kept secret. Both keys are required to decrypt a message.

smart card. a card about the size of a credit card that carries an electronic memory of such items as patient records or user authentication information.

strong encryption. highly sophisticated encryption techniques that use very large, often prime, numbers in the algorithms. Strong encryption is recommended for transmission of highly secure information.

virtual private network. the use of encryption to provide a secure connection through an insecure network such as the Internet.

REFERENCES

Davis, B. (1997, September 8). Security survey: Is it safe? *Information Week.*

Heath, J. (1997–1998). *How electronic encryption works and how it will change your business.* Available: http://www.viacorp.com/crypto.html

Kabay, M.E. (1998). *ICSA white paper on crime statistics.* International Computer Security Association. Available: http://www.icsa.net/library/research/comp_crime.shtml

Network Authentication Solutions: Who knows who you are? Infoworld. Available: http://www.infoworld.com/cgi-bin/displayTC.pl?/970616comp.htm

Romney, Steinbart, & Cushing (1997). *Accounting information systems* (7th ed.). Reading, MA: Addison-Wesley.

Smith, S. (1998). *Top 10 technology opportunities: Tips and tools.* Sarasota, FL: American Institute of Public Accountants.

Winkler, I. (1997). *Why hackers do the things they do.* International Computer Security Association. Available: http://www.icsa.net/library/research/i.shtml

CHAPTER 16

Information Technology

Robert H. Jackson, Jr.

TABLE OF CONTENTS

EXECUTIVE SUMMARY

Informunication—the fusion of information and communication—is creating new opportunities and demands for today's physician leaders. Our fast–paced culture of change necessitates critical changes in public leadership style through mastery of collaborative partnerships and goal-focused change brokering, while managing the emerging information and communication-driven business enterprise. Personal lifelong learning methods incorporating new research processes, just-in-time learning opportunities, and assessment of trends are necessary to strengthen physician's critical knowledge bases. Adaptation to these new demands requires a practical and sustainable implementation plan including specific technology skills needed by successful physician leaders.

FIGHTING AGAINST THE FUTURE

The cardinal returned this spring.

I paused bleary eyed in the living room doorway one spring morning to a strange thumping sound—not rhythmic, but with a certain slow and annoying regularity. As he had done hundreds, perhaps thousands of times last year, a male cardinal flung itself against the solid glass french doors to my deck. Hidden just out of eyesight at the edge of the room, I watched it first perch on the top of my iron deck chairs, tilting its head left and right, ruffling its feathers, and cocking its head, again staring directly in the plate glass. Then suddenly, it would fly—full force—into the glass, fiercely attacking its mate's supposed suitor. Momentarily stunned by the force of the blow as he hit the glass, he fell and just caught himself in flight before hitting my deck. Leaping back to his iron seat-back perch, he began again a long stare at the glass.

For hours every day throughout this spring as he had done the year before, this crazy bird would repeat the sequence—sit, tilt, ruffle, tilt, attack, fall, and return to sit again. His muted gray mate would sometimes perch a short distance away on the lawn furniture and watch the proceedings—sometimes not. No matter to the defending male—he planned to conquer this stubborn and strong foe with his own tenacity.

Little did he know that his spouse's vying young suitor was nothing more than his own reflection in the shiny glass.

Many of us are like this bird. Convinced that the enemy is just ahead, we muster every ounce of energy and frantically, repeatedly throw ourselves and our thoughts and our careers at the beast in our path. But the beast is unwavering. And unhurt. We fail to see that the beast we fight is a creation of our own minds.

A Culture of Change for Individuals and Businesses

Our culture of change continues its frantic pace. New technology creates whole new markets overnight—and just as rapidly collapses them. Netscape Communications single-handedly created an entirely new market of point-and-click web browsers to service a relatively unknown Internet communications hypertext transfer protocol (HTTP) and now struggles to retain any market share of its original product segment (Gimein, 1998). Apple Computer not only created the personal computer in the late 1970s, but it pioneered computer graphics-based user interfaces in its Macintosh. Today, Apple sees its hardware market share and mind share a mere shadow of its former self and its graphic concepts incorporated into rival machines that outsell its own twenty to one (Kanellos, 1997).

Change is not confined to the technology arena only. Stockbrokers struggle with whole new classes of investors (including mutual fund managers and Internet-connected individuals) who are less willing to pay premium brokerages fees for basic stock transaction services. Parents wrestle with the paradox of 500 available cable channels and very little appropriate entertainment content for their children. And an entirely new universe of American-branded managed medical care systems has turned physician, patient, and insurer relationships upside down.

Our world moves quickly

Try as we might, today's breakneck speed of change is unlikely to slow. For to slow would require a shrinkage in business climate, pace of progress, and volume of progressive research and application knowledge. Indeed, an accurate, quantitative measure of the rate of change in all cultural, political, technical, and economic segments would be a strong predictor in the overall well being of businesses, countries, and indeed our world, rivaling even our ponderous official government indexes in accuracy.

Such a comprehensive measure of "info-flation" does not currently exist. And that is just as well, since an accurate assessment of the increasing amount and speed of communication and information it conveys might emotionally overwhelm a significant population segment—perhaps friends and coworkers. Perhaps ourselves.

Still, ours is a culture of change. And a culture we must face daily. Shall we fling ourselves vainly against plate glass fighting virtual wars and encountering barriers made of our own minds? Can we beat more time out of the same twenty-four hour day? Or can we learn to work smarter, not harder?

INFORMUNICATION

The war is born of change. Our best response is found in adapting to change. Embracing a change-tolerant paradigm—or more simply, a new series of personal habits—not only keeps us from fighting imaginary wars with change but equips us to battle in the language of change so critical to our success.

We live in an era some have called the Information Age. That phrase may be shortsighted and is certainly incomplete. Information has always been with us. It is the powerful, synergistic combination of information and communication that propels today's world. Let us call this new paradigm—this new thinking and action process—Informunication. Informunication can be defined as the use of technology-leveraged, knowledge-focused collaboration systems to inform, empower, and advance individuals and organizations. Business, politics, power and culture all are now deeply influenced—for better or worse—by our new "Informunication Age."

Two new basic skills are required in this age of Informunication. Your personal approach to formal and informal leadership must adapt. So must your commitment to learning.

NEW BASIC SKILLS: A CHANGE IN LEADERSHIP APPROACH

Collaborative Partnerships

Leadership in the Informunication Age faces a significant change in functional style. No longer the absolute monarch of an industry, today's business leader must become the master of collaborative partnerships. History teaches us that countries selecting economic isolationism (the political equal of industry monarch) eventually collapse in upon themselves

(Schlesinger, 1952). In less tasteful terms, singular personality-driven enterprises create a kind of business incest, which fails to refresh the economic and energetic bloodline of an enterprise. Sure, it is a short, heady trip in self-esteem to be recognized as "The One" for whom the business stands. But it is the vitality, risk sharing, and the subtle, incalculable value of synergy and partnering in a mutually beneficial cause which accounts for ongoing success. Look carefully into history to find that the most successful and longest-lived leadership dynasties were and remain those leaders whose ability to partner and collaborate shines above all else. They possessed the uncanny knack to gather high-caliber people around a mutually shared goal.

Change Brokering

Leadership will also become more a process of successfully brokering change towards business advantage. Henry Ford didn't create either the assembly line or the automobile. But Ford recognized a sea change, took tools others had developed, and produced a product the customer wanted. Nothing particularly special about what he did, except that he brokered an impending change to his advantage. Change brokers—those who go beyond mere visionaries and develop practical change manipulation skills—will drive tomorrow's economy.

The Informunication-driven Enterprise

Leadership in the Informunication Age must also create an information and communication-driven enterprise. What are the characteristics of your best clients? Of your worst? How long do your best clients stick with you? How variable is that statistic? What product or services in your business has the best margin? Which has the worst? Has anyone ever made money on the item or service that gives you the lowest margin? The answers to these questions should be readily accessible in real time to a physician leader invested in an informunication-savvy enterprise. Savvy extends beyond having the latest PCs and the newest analytical software. Savvy involves a ground-level commitment to asking proactive, business-centric questions and monitoring progress as an integrated operating principle. Sophisticated electronic performance support systems (EPSS) are beginning to develop a robust, well-rounded technical foundation for management decision processes by summary analysis of daily—sometimes hourly—business pulse points in a clear, easily absorbed presentation (*A learning page for EPPS,* 1997).

NEW BASIC SKILLS: A COMMITMENT TO LIFELONG LEARNING

Successful business professionals in the Informunication Age will also show strong personal commitment to lifelong learning. Learning no longer is a specific event or a process constrained between two dates of a calendar or the hands of a clock. Learning must become a lifelong process.

New Research Methods

New methods and modalities of research will accompany lifelong learning. Are you aware that the encyclopedia is obsolete? Internet search engines not only can present the same factual information once found in our 26 volume bound editions, but can link directly to subjects in today's up-to-the-minute headlines. Need to know something about your competition? Check them out on the web. Competent on-line research skills are a requisite personal skill in today's business. Knowing how to narrow an on-line search from keywords with 20,000 "hits" to just the three most relevant for your review is a practical skill you may have missed in earlier schooling, yet cannot afford to miss in tomorrow's world.

Just-in-Time Learning

Just-in-time learning will progress from an education form reserved for trade skills to an accepted and requisite environment for professionals in all areas. Combined with dexterity in on-line research, you can refresh yourself daily in areas where information expands faster than your ability to casually absorb and retain. Compare your diagnosis with others on-line or leave a question with an on-line discussion group and get the answer in a few hours from experts in the field.

Trend Spotting

Successful lifelong learners in the Informunication Age will develop a valuable sixth sense for spotting trends. Trend spotting might include the ability to expect specific technology innovations or a sense for the effect on global markets in the face of regional economic events. Such a knowledge-based skill is not new—successful stockbrokers and technology leaders have been spotting trends as a profession for many years. However, trend spotting is now a logical and critically important application of the knowledge lifelong learners will be acquiring. As more and more people develop this previously rare ability to gather and assess raw knowledge, accurate and timely trend spotting will become a basic skill set. Failure to predict a significant range of such trends will lead to business and financial reversals far more quickly in the near future than in the past. Previously, knowledge-based trend spotting was rare and generally resulted in isolated millionaires (such as Apple's Stephen Jobs and Lotus' Mitch Kapor). Today, however, information once scarce and slow-moving is now more broadly available. More people will be able to detect and respond to emerging trends. Isolated financial successes will likely be harder to come by. Those without these assessment skills may no longer survive their passive stance. Failure to actively forecast in response to trends will quickly diminish opportunity for market share or competitive advantage.

THE URGENCY OF ADAPTATION

Making a personal and professional commitment in this Informunication Age has become an urgent and time-sensitive requirement. Adaptation of your personal lifestyle to the new basic skill sets of change-brokering leadership and lifelong learning likely requires a significant and nontrivial adjustment in everything from your daily schedule to your use of financial resources.

Two guidelines may be useful in adapting personally and professionally to this culture of change and the requirements of the Informunication Age. First, select appropriate technology as your first-line tool set for adaptation. Second, when implementing technology or informunication-related systems, be cautious, though not necessarily slow, in its roll-out.

Technology as a Tool, Not a Toy

Appropriately used in business and professional endeavors, technology is a tool, not a toy. Many of us are or know people surrounded by gadgets—indoor golf putters, wireless built-in CD players, desktop noisemakers that produce a random stream of yes, no, and maybe as a decision support tool. These are things that entertain and amuse, things that are cool and trendy, but in the end, they are nothing more than things and gadgets. Computers and communication systems can be among those gadgets accumulated in life but attracting nothing more than dust. Possession of garden shears does not make you a productive gardener—it is the skill borne of experience and dedication with which you plant and use nurturing shears to trim and prune that determines your value with the tool.

Implementation as a River, Not a Waterfall

Implementation plans should be treated as rivers, not waterfalls. Do not expect a revolutionary process for incorporating new tools into your personal or professional activities to be met with open arms by your associates. Be evolutionary, not revolutionary, in introducing adaptive and change-anticipatory technology systems. Humans and computers interact in complex ways and their relationship is constantly in flux. Early in the Information Age, this interaction required arcane programming skills tailored to machine architectures and failed to address the variety and styles of output most meaningful to we humans. Fortunately, market-driven forces of capitalism have rewarded client-focused technology developers who refine computer operations to more closely match expected human norms. Better software techniques constantly improve our ability to input and extract information in meaningful ways without having to immerse ourselves in programming or other complex "technobable." Seek always to develop technology plans that emphasize the cultural and personality-driven nuances of our workplaces and equip them with tools of appropriate technology. Understand that knowledge gained is productively used only by people committed to positive change.

Critical Technology Skills for Personal Adaptation

Personal implementation plans begin with a frank assessment of the technology skills critical to successful physician leaders. Personal computing has revolutionized the way individuals collect, organize, and store information. Familiarity with word processing, a skill once reserved for clerks and junior staff, has become a mandatory personal skill in this informunication age for both personal note taking and the email-enabled communications that bypass old-fashioned telephone tag for the crispness, clarity, and speed. The ability to personally manage and critically analyze electronic spreadsheets, research, and collaborate interactively over the web using digital voice–integrated, graphics-intensive data presentation are all key skills in creating a persuasive process and presentation. How many of these crucial skills are in your personal skill set today?

CONCLUSION

Many of us fling ourselves against the plate glass in frustration—trying to win a battle formed of our own minds while missing today's real business battles all together. Information communicated—informunication—may help us successfully adapt to changes already alive in our personal and professional environments. An executive MBA program should equip you for this sea change—teaching technology and Internet communication skills to help you confidently take the helm. Searching the web, using Powerpoint to make persuasive presentations, building analytical graphics from your spreadsheet—all these skills should progress from science fiction to way of life in your professional portfolio.

The Informunication Age is dawning. Are you ready?

GLOSSARY

http. hyper text transfer protocol. a protocol used on the Internet to allow computers to request and receive information. The technical foundation of the World Wide Web.

informunication. a coined term describing the use of technology-leveraged knowledge-focused collaboration systems to inform, empower, and advance individuals and organizations.

internet. a globally available communications system interconnecting computers and the information on them. Available to consumers with a wide range of costs, speeds, and value added.

proactive. anticipatory action; being ahead of the game.

synergy. In the context of relationships, the effect of producing more or better results through collaboration or partnerships than could be achieved through the summation of individuals.

web browser. software allowing access to major portions of the Internet through graphical and easy-to-use computer displays.

REFERENCES

Gimein, M. (1998). Netscape browser share continues to fall. *The Industry Standard* [on-line]. Available: http://www.idg.net/idg_frames/english/content.cgi?vc=docid_9-65044.html (Accessed November, 1998).

Kanellos, M. (1997). Apple market share sinks again. CNET NEWS.COM [on-line]. Available: http://www.news.com/News/Item/0,4,17293,00.html (Accessed November, 1998).

A learning page for EPSS (1997). [on-line]. Available: http://train.ed.psu.edu/learner/epss/ (Accessed November, 1998).

Schlesinger, A.M., Jr. (1952). The new isolationism. *The Atlantic Monthly, 189*(5), 34–38.

Index